DEAR DOCTOR

DEAR DOCTOR

WHAT DOCTORS DON'T ASK,
WHAT PATIENTS NEED TO SAY

MARILYN McENTYRE

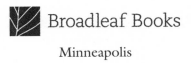

Broadleaf Books

Minneapolis

DEAR DOCTOR
What Doctors Don't Ask, What Patients Need to Say

Cover design: Lindsey Owens
Cover photo: XiXinXing/iStock

Print ISBN: 978-1-5064-6047-5
eBook ISBN: 978-1-5064-6048-2

For Guy Micco and for the Writers
in the UCB-UCSF Joint Medical Program,
with admiration and gratitude.

TABLE OF CONTENTS

INTRODUCTION

The concerns that take us to doctors vary widely. Some of them, as we have witnessed daily in months of pandemic, are emergency situations. Triage. Others are the more "ordinary" annual checkups, standard visits for routine tests or minor ailments—or when we suspect something more concerning might be amiss. In those visits we begin to understand how important it is to frame and ask real questions that may not be on intake questionnaires—or on the table, until we put them there. This book is for those times, which are never, for the sick, "ordinary."

JUST FILL OUT THIS form and the nurse will call you in a few minutes." We put down name, address, age, gender, insurance number, and emergency contact. We check boxes, three columns of them, scanning through a list of the most common diseases known to North Americans. We're given three or four lines on which to explain our check marks: "Shoulder pain continues from an old tennis injury." "I control diabetes with diet." "Severe monthly cramps since early adolescence." And so on. Then we page through old issues of *People* magazine, if we're desperate for diversion, and wait.

Once we're ushered into an examination room, we put on the paper gown, gaze at posters featuring major muscle groups or the alimentary canal, and fiddle with our phones. At long last, the doctor knocks politely, walks in, perhaps clutching a laptop, and we begin.

A focused, practical, and kindly conversation most likely ensues. Even in overcrowded and understaffed urban offices, I've met with doctors who are uncommonly open-hearted and manage to convey authentic concern about even minor ailments in the ten to twelve minutes available. My observation, after years of regular visits ranging from routine checkups to a few surgeries, is that most people who go into clinical medicine are compassionate and humane—if also harried, hurried, and occasionally sleep-deprived. They work under considerable constraints: keeping records, managing the office, staying abreast of new regulations and software, reading lab reports, attending professional conferences, and interpreting test data, take more of their time than most of us realize. Some of them mentor medical students. Some volunteer in free clinics for the growing number of people without adequate housing or medical care. They want to be healers. And most of us who go see them want more than a prescription. We want to be healed. For some of us, this involves changing deeply entrenched habits, becoming more aware of the ways we participate in social and corporate systems that affect public health, and learning to change our notions of "normal." We'd like a little more from these medical professionals who are already stretched, stressed, and sometimes squashed into institutional schedules that don't allow much time for visiting. Still, I don't think I'm alone in wishing those visits to be more exploratory, humane, widely focused on the contexts in which we try to maintain health and wholeness, especially when those contexts involve social or economic marginalization.

In addition to clinical encounters for my own health concerns, I've had the privilege of working with medical students, premed students, and students entering other health care professions for over twenty years. Some were children of doctors, groomed and eager to follow parents who had modeled a love of medicine. Some were children of immigrant farmworkers, the first in their families to attend college, eager to return to under-served communities and help provide more adequate health care. Some were students who had struggled with chronic illness or disability themselves, entering medicine a little more familiar than most with the view from the hospital bed. Some had cared for dying parents, or volunteered in a clinic, or traveled on medical mission trips, or donated platelets to a sibling. One had consigned her daughter's vital organs to several unknown recipients after a fatal accident.

Knowing these people has immensely enriched my teaching life and, more importantly, my sense of what health care can and should mean. Witnessing clinicians at work has given me a deep appreciation for the generosity, imagination, and life-giving curiosities that lead people into a demanding profession they know will cost them sleep; expose them to pathogens and to people's pain, grief, and tears; and enmesh them in a beleaguered bureaucratic system riddled with political tensions and insurance forms.

I've also had the privilege of working alongside professors and doctors who usher those students through anatomy and physiology, and clinical skills. Among them are people whose compassion has been a beacon for me, as well as for those they teach. They've given me glimpses of medicine "from the inside."

I do not have a medical degree; my training is in literature and language. Medicine was my "road not taken." But teaching American literature opened a back door into medicine. Questions about illness, injury, disability, dying, and human suffering inevitably came up in English courses, even as we made our way through *Moby-Dick*, *The Sound and the Fury*, and *Bless Me, Ultima*. Illness, injury, disability, and death are part of every human story. The stories every culture inscribes and passes on are largely about how people cope.

Through stories—both fictional and true—written by people with illness or disability and those who cared for them, I was led to new questions about diagnosis, treatment, medical authority, public health problems, and patients' predicaments. I read about abuse and trauma from survivors who'd had to find a path through almost unimaginable horrors. As I read first *The Bluest Eye* and later *Beloved*, I felt grateful for Toni Morrison's unflinching courage in helping readers imagine how abuse happens and is perpetuated, even as I recoiled from the horrors she recounts. I read twentieth-century poets who helped readers imagine diabetes, cancer, and bipolar disorder in ways that foster deeper compassion for people living with those conditions. I read plays written at the height of the AIDS epidemic that were comic, tragic, enraging, sobering, and disturbing.

Imagine my delight when, a few decades ago, I discovered "medical humanities," which is a field of study concerned with the cultural dimensions of medical practice, i.e., the role of story-making in clinical encounters—for instance, the way language choices, especially metaphors, shape practical decisions in health care; what poetry by patients can teach us about pain; and how reflective writing can help practitioners engage with their own uncertainties, sorrows, irritations, anxieties, and perspective.

Ever since teaching my first course on "Medicine in Literature," I've enjoyed being in hospitals and the halls of medical schools, talking with clinicians over coffee, or interviewing patient-poets, or finding my own path into patient care as a hospice volunteer, or sometimes as a patient—curious even when I was in pain about how healing may happen.

That enjoyment led me to write this book. I'm writing it as an open letter to a doctor to invite not only medical professionals, but also everyone who visits them, to make our conversations about health and well-being more useful by making them more reflective, inclusive, and relational. I hope my musings will help both doctors and patients widen the clinical conversation, even within its stringent time constraints, to consider information likely overlooked or excluded during routine data gathering.

Good doctors understand the medical relevance of a patient's food preferences, spiritual practices, and what news they watch. But questions about any of those can remain unasked on a scheduled visit when time is short and the waiting room is full. The time primary-care physicians have to spend with each patient is, in most contemporary medical settings in the US, severely limited; depending on the setting, visits with doctors in most insurance networks range from five to twenty-five minutes and include frequent interruptions. But in those minutes, doctors are able to touch patients in ways no one else can. In addition to writing out prescriptions, they ask about intimate matters that would be no one else's business, offer advice and reminders we may know but need to hear (and perhaps can't hear from those nearest to us at home), and deliver news that sometimes changes us forever.

Even though I've devoted whole chapters to matters that deserve more "air time" in conversations between doctors and patients, I'm not imagining any of us will enjoy the luxury of ninety-minute office visits. Still, as

I've explored these areas of concern, I've repeatedly recalled the question a medical school professor asked the interns she trained: "If you had two extra minutes with a patient, what would you do with them?"

This question forces those interns, already involved in patient care, to pause and consider how they inhabit time, how they budget it, and how they might bring fuller attention to the moments they have with those for whom they care. Sometimes those extra moments—those two minutes—might save a life, allowing for something withheld out of reticence or dread to emerge and be addressed.

Try this: set your timer and sit in silence for two whole minutes just to realize how long they are. As you read these chapters, think about those two minutes. Think about how one question clearly asked and one answer thoughtfully—albeit briefly—articulated, might change your and your doctor's approach to the work of healing, and help make healing happen.

Sometimes, those who offer us prescription drugs are frustrated because they would also like to offer healing presence, comfort, attention, and informed encouragement. The promise of being healers led them into medicine. Healing work takes time, imagination, personal engagement, awareness of how mind, emotions, values, and language affect the life of the body. Even acknowledging those dimensions of illness and health can enhance a person's resilience. There's good reason to believe most of us barely tap the resources available to us in reflection, meditation, prayer, conscious eating, or simple conversation as we navigate the rough waters of occasional, chronic, or terminal illness.

I wrote this book as a letter to a doctor, having in mind several good ones I am grateful to have witnessed at work. The "Dear Doctor" I address is one who listens deeply and thoughtfully, wants to keep learning, reflects with an open heart, and cultivates lively curiosity informed by humility.

I hope this book equips both patients and doctors with strategies for more life-giving conversations, however brief they may be—the kind of conversations Jesus invited when he asked the lame man, "Do you want to be healed?" It's not an idle question. We all have reason to consider it and to find hope in the fact that grace and growth can happen swiftly and suddenly if we make room.

AN AWKWARD ARRANGEMENT

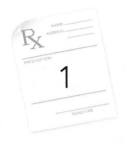

Shame can be exacerbated or even incited by physicians through judgment and as a result of the power imbalance inherent to the physician-patient dynamic, compounded by the contemporary tendency to moralise about "lifestyle" illnesses.

—LUNA DOLEZAL

I will remember that there is art to medicine as well as science, and that warmth, sympathy, and understanding may outweigh the surgeon's knife or the chemist's drug.

—2019 VERSION OF THE HIPPOCRATIC OATH

I KNOW YOU HAVE OTHER patients waiting. I know you need to know my weight. I know you've seen hundreds of private body parts. And I know you do this every day. But I don't. I don't like disrobing and sitting, cold and mottled, on a strip of paper with bare feet dangling, while you stand nearby, dignified and professional in your white coat, and ask questions. I don't like mentioning the "unmentionable" (bowel movements, urinary habits, sex). No matter how much we normalize this situation, it's a long leap from most social guidelines about modesty and polite discretion to the kinds of humiliating exposure your medical questions and touching and tests require. So I guess we need to talk about tact, the inherent social awkwardness of an office visit, and how empathy can make the sudden necessity of "indecent exposure" more tolerable.

I read an article recently that claimed nearly all physicians believed patients lied or omitted facts. I imagine most of us do find ways to dodge the uncomfortable parts of an already embarrassing conversation—the parts about age spots and sagging breasts, or how much we actually drink after a hard day at work, or about constipation or gas or other matters we may not even talk about with our life partners. The writer who reported the frequency of patients' lies (or, let's say, evasions or half-conscious deceptions) made one fact startlingly plain: "Many Americans say they would rather live in pain than visit their doctor." That seems like a sad commentary on the celebrated efforts to teach medical students how to "partner" with patients, but I can understand why patients flee. Or procrastinate. I certainly have. I'm overdue for a few "routine" tests even as we speak. Because I, like many others, find it challenging to talk with complete candor about my body.

I remember reading with a shock of recognition Lucy Pearce's observation in *Medicine Woman* that most of us "have grown up feeling alienated in our bodies, embarrassed or ashamed of them, not at home in our physical selves." I still remember, sometimes painfully, long moments of relentless self-scrutiny in front of the mirror before leaving for school, acutely aware of every pimple and freckle and fat deposit. I think how painfully it may apply to people who have to endure forms of social marginalization that often get internalized as debilitating self-judgment. Pearce goes on to say, "[We] have internalized the message that there's something wrong with us, rather than there is something wrong." That sentence hit me hard; I realized how quickly and reflexively I may complicate whatever "straightforward" problem we're discussing with guilt, or shame, or self-judgment. Those feelings become inhibiting factors in our office visits. Atul Gawande, another medical writer who kept me happily paying for a *New Yorker* subscription for many months, commented with characteristic elegance and empathy on the self-defeating messages we patients bring into the office, clinic, and hospital:

> We're always trotting out some story of a ninety-seven-year-old who runs marathons, as if such cases were not miracles of biological luck but [rather] reasonable expectations for all. Then, when our bodies fail to live up to this fantasy, we feel as if we somehow have something to apologize for.

I have my equivalent of that ninety-seven-year-old runner. She's a pain. She and the Inner Critic are frequent unwelcome, uninvited guests who follow me to the mirror every time I brush my graying hair. They and I walk into your office knowing we're part of a culture that makes health and longevity a moral virtue, and therefore implicitly assigns blame for many health problems by suggesting those problems are simply a function of bad personal choices. We have been conditioned in subtle and not-so-subtle ways to associate sickness or debility with moral weakness, or at least lack of gumption or grit.

So many of us walk into your office feeling a little defective or vaguely at fault for being sick.

Because I've hung around medical schools for a while, teaching the not-really-medicine courses students occasionally take (that involve, to the surprise of the more hard-core scientific types among them, stories and poems), I know the best of those schools have been trying for at least a decade to create a place for reflection, empathy, compassion, and emotional sensitivity within each doctor's practice. I'm encouraged to see that coaching on communication skills and styles is happening in medical education all over the country. Did you come from a medical program that has begun to require "specific instruction and evaluation of [communication] skills . . . including communication with patients, families, colleagues and other health professionals"? Or have you attended professional workshops with that focus? I hope so. Apparently, they promote measurably greater "patient satisfaction."

Since your profession requires you to deliver unwelcome information in uncomfortable settings to reluctant recipients who often come with unrealistic hopes for cures or solutions, "satisfaction" may be hard to achieve.

Some groups that study patient satisfaction represent patients like me as "consumers" or "customers." But I don't consider myself a consumer or customer when

I'm shivering on that examining table. Yes, the matter of money is never completely off the table (more about that later); what insurance will pay for always matters. So, in that sense, I'm a consumer. But the satisfaction I look for is a comfortable certainty that I can trust you, your professional judgments, your personal integrity, your interest in my case, your willingness and capacity to be in the moment (or the few moments) we have together without distraction, and your investment in my well-being. Good medicine is relational. Even when, at some point, you or some other doctor tells me I'm not likely to recover—and I imagine that day will come—I hope I can be satisfied that whatever must be said will be handled with honesty, clarity, attention, and care.

"Empathy" may be a lot to hope for; it is much more intimate and emotionally demanding than sympathy. But I do expect imagination and tact. I expect you to do what you can to alleviate the unavoidable unease of our having to talk about delicate or disagreeable things in settings that are inherently disempowering for me. This disempowerment often begins with the shedding of my clothing. I recall a friend of mine acknowledging his resistance to simple checkups, commenting, "I remember a recent visit when the nurse said, 'Strip down to your shorts. The doctor will be right in,' after which I waited in an unnecessarily chilly room for ten or fifteen minutes, shivering and unnecessarily underclad." Even the word "strip" is jarring. His story made me aware of three simple things I expect when I come to see you: appropriately dignified language, reasonable temperature, and realistic time estimates (a five- or six-minute wait isn't "a moment"). And, of course, I expect respect, even as you're having to instruct me to change my indulgent habits, or delivering health advice I've known and ignored for decades, or urging me somehow to get a grip and try harder.

I know what I'm suggesting is not always simple. Bridging the gaps that divide you doctors from the rest of us by class, professional status, and sometimes gender is never simple. As a woman who has given birth three times, I am aware, for instance, of how sometimes comic, as well as disconcerting, it is when men try to coach women through childbirth. My obstetricians, for reasons then beyond my control, were all men. A passage in Ree Drummond's *The Pioneer Woman* comes to mind as I recall those experiences:

> "Go ahead and push once for me," Dr. Oliver said.
>
> I did, but only hard enough to ensure that nothing accidental or embarrassing would slip out. I could think of no greater humiliation.

7

"Okay, that's not going to work at all," Dr. Oliver scolded.

I pushed again.

"Ree," Dr. Oliver said, looking up at me through the space between my legs. "You can do way better than that."

Despite the wry note the writer strikes in this scene, it's hard not to hear "for me" as infantilizing and "scolded" as odiously paternalistic.

When I find myself in conversations about the importance of empathy in medical care, I take the word "empathy" to mean an ability (and willingness) to imagine patients' pain, sorrow, fear, resistance, rage, or hope. I take it also to mean a certain deftness at offsetting the clumsiness and power differential in those moments of unequal vulnerability between us. That kind of skillful, practical empathy requires maturity and training. I'd like you to know how much I appreciate any effort you make to be empathetic, compassionate, and tactful when you're required to trespass into private territory. I appreciate small acknowledgments of what is necessarily uncomfortable, such as, "I'm aware it may be difficult to talk about this, but . . ." or "If you feel comfortable telling me a bit more, I'd like to know . . ." I appreciate your respecting me as a peer, especially when I'm feeling disempowered, subordinated, naked, and cold.

If we're going to get through the awkwardness to a place of honesty and ease, we need to do a certain amount of trust building. I need to trust your discretion. I need to feel assured that nothing about what transpires in the exam room will become an amusing story in the doctors' break room, that my capacity to understand possible side effects or an explanation of treatment options won't be underestimated. That my anxieties, even if baseless, won't be dismissed, or glossed over, or patted down.

It's unsettling to find myself in a one-down position with another adult professional. I imagine I'm not that different from other patients who have had to rearrange their demanding schedules to fit yours. We all know that's a practical necessity. For the poorer among us, it is very likely a hardship. But part of my discomfort that comes from stepping out of my "territory" into yours is the feeling of sudden infantilization. My fears are exposed, just like my body parts, and yours aren't. My anxieties about what "routine" tests will show, or about the impact of my health concerns (and medical expenses) on my family, or about how my work life may have to change, or my food habits are all a little embarrassing. "Routine" isn't a convincing word. These things are not routine for me. I'm not

Patient X. I need to hear language that opens room for questions—even the occasional explicit invitations to ask questions—about terms, or statistical possibilities, or biological processes. I need help imagining what's taking place under (or on) my skin without being made to feel I'm wasting your valuable time. And I need the answers not to be dumbed down, though they may need to be brief.

One of the most memorable portrayals I've seen of awkward clinical encounters is in Margaret Edson's play, *W;t* (1995). Emma Thompson's leading role in its cable television movie adaptation (2001) is extraordinary. I urge you to see it! In it, an aging English professor, herself inclined to an attitude of snobbish intellectual superiority, is treated by a celebrated research oncologist whose deficiency in human kindness undermines his impressive credentials. His assistant happens to be an intern who was once a hapless student in the patient's English class. Although the situation itself has broad comedic possibilities and the dialogue is laced with dry wit at its best, the deepest note of *W;t* is one of pathos. What the patient most needs, even though she is unable to acknowledge it until the end, is tenderness. Her human, even childlike, needs are met best when a sympathetic nurse, in the end stages of her care as she nears death, brings her a Popsicle and an old teacher reads her a children's story about the runaway bunny whose mother will find her no matter where she goes. She needs to hear that message: *You are loved. You are safe in that love. You will be brought home.* It is a word of spiritual comfort that reaches across traditions to address the fears that come with human vulnerability and mortality.

While I can't imagine a situation in which you would (or in which I would want you to) sit down and read me *The Runaway Bunny*, I can imagine a bold allusion to those stories. Stories are sources of deep reassurance for us—Biblical tales of healing and restoration; myths about injury and recovery, or abandonment and finding; or profiles in courage. Literature, film, and music—from the Psalms to Tibetan chant to Judy Garland belting out "Over the Rainbow"—offer a huge repertoire of comforting words and images. Some of them soothingly play in our heads in time of need. Though it won't likely be you, I hope someone will be nearby to read, or sing, or just hum a bit to soften what is very hard when I'm in great pain, or languishing in a long recovery, or facing death.

It's cheering to know more and more medical schools are offering some training in the humanities and arts because they're a fundamental—not just elective— dimension of clinical training. One young doctor wrote about this kind of training in a 2016 *New York Times* article that testified to the value of what he learned from an art history course in medical school:

> The purpose was to help us become more thoughtful and meticulous observers—a skill, perhaps more than any other, that lays the foundation for good medicine.
>
> In the coming months, the class's lessons would creep up on me at unexpected moments during patient rounds: noting asymmetry on an old man's face; describing angry purple blisters to a colleague; considering the shadowy contours of pneumonia on an X-ray.

Awareness of this kind enlarges one's capacity to care. It fosters the empathy that dispels awkwardness. Attentiveness is deep, generous attention—not just prolonged. It is sharper, and kinder, and more curious. To gaze at a portrait, or to read a poem, or to hit replay to hear a musical passage again cultivates the "deep, sustained, undeviating" attention that musician Roberto Gerhard describes as "an experience of a very high order."

It matters to me to know you've paused over an image of Michelangelo's *Pietà* to take in a mother's sorrow; or seen the deepening shadow of mental illness in Van Gogh's late self-portraits; or thought about how community copes with disability and epidemic illness as you gazed at the jarring varieties of human suffering in Bruegel's *Fight Between Carnival and Lent*, or registered something new about horror when you first looked at Munch's *The Scream*—a face that forces us to feel, if just for a moment, the scope of the horrors that have unfolded among us in the past two centuries. It would strengthen my confidence in your capacity to help me through whatever I have to face if I knew you had listened to (or played, or sung) a Bach cantata or been moved by Bessie Griffin singing "Sometimes I Feel Like a Motherless Child." I'd like to know phrases from poetry and song and story might be shared reference points that connect my suffering with others' when it's my turn.

I'd like to challenge you to meet me on that ground occasionally. Even as you challenge me to take care of my fitness and general health, I'd like you to read enough good books, see enough good movies, or watch enough sporting events to recognize references to them when they arise and allow them to pave over that bumpy, unmapped, empty space between us. Finding those points of contact is the best way I know to get beyond awkward and drop into a deeper awareness of what we share as human beings—vulnerability, curiosity, the need for kindness and honesty, respect, and the genuine attention that says, "I see you. I care. Let's walk this diffi-cult stretch of the journey together. Let's find things out. And let's remind each other in those two minutes we might have of a scene, or image, or music that may bring a moment of life-giving energy, comic relief, or solidarity into the space between us.

My Two Minutes: What have you learned about tact in the examining room? How do you get past your own inhibitions about seeing and touching other people's bodies? How do you think about "professionalism"?

In It Together

> True patient-centered care requires providers
> and practices to forge strong partnerships with
> patients and families.
> —Agency for Healthcare Research and Quality

THE DOCTORS WHO HAVE helped me most have asked
surprising questions: *What color is your headache? What
happens when you laugh? How are you like your mother?
What are you holding onto that you might need to let go?*
They have also, in addition to occasional antibiotics or
pain relievers, given me suggestions I suspect didn't
come from medical textbooks: *Assume pain is a message
and see if you can learn what your body has to tell you.
Eat red things.* And my favorite: *Go outside at night and*

spend two minutes gazing at the moon. (Try this. Something shifts.)

These startling questions and suggestions came from medical doctors, not therapists. They emerged during conventional inquiries about sleep patterns, intensity and location of pain, genetics, onset of the last period, elimination habits, and stress. Most of the conversations I have in doctors' offices are brief and strictly focused on symptoms or, as medical students learn to put it, the "history of present illness." But I've learned that information I might once not have mentioned can be more relevant than I realize. I've also learned that the doctors who help me the most reserve a few minutes for whatever miscellany might emerge in response to the general query, "What else is going on?"

So, dear doctor, I'm writing to see if we can help each other make better use of our ten to fifteen minutes together. I'm not out to reform medicine, but rather to inform the medical professionals I rely on that there are things I could tell you that might provide missing pieces in a puzzle if you asked the right questions. And there are questions I might ask if I felt they would be welcomed and taken seriously. Some of those questions might open doors to a deeper understanding of illness, pain, suffering, or fatigue.

Because I spend some of my work life with medical professionals, I've had a chance to notice a shift in the language some doctors use about their work over the years. Instead of "treating patients," some prefer to talk about "partnering with patients"—a phrase that sounds refreshingly egalitarian to a layperson like me who has often felt disempowered by brisk (or brusque) people in white coats. "Partnering" reminds me that I bring something to the table that can help us both work better together. It's not a new idea: one doctor I know likes to quote a nineteenth-century physician, William Osler, who famously advised his students, "Just listen to your patient. He is telling you the diagnosis." Listening is hard. It requires sustained eye contact, taking your hands off the keyboard, and not thinking about your next patient. Or lunch.

As a new patient, I'm hoping you're a doctor who, without irony, thinks of healing work as a partnership. I hope when I walk into your office, you see me as someone who knows things about her body, her emotions, and herself that may help you help me. I hope you see my health issues as having a unique history. I hope you consider how that history happened in a tangled web of family culture, mass marketing, and inherited, unexamined notions about health and illness.

I hope you remember patients like me are inhibited when we're scared of symptoms, intimidated by white coats, and disinclined to ask questions. I read the story of one doctor, also a breast cancer survivor, who acknowledged how difficult it was to have a thorough, clear, and informative conversation during a crisis since the whole subject of chemotherapy was "clearly overwhelming" in the immediate wake of a dire diagnosis. "It became rather difficult," she wrote, "to explain the principles of chemotherapy in the level of detail I would have wanted had we only more time with patients." I will return later to the problem of severe time constraints that determine the way we communicate. The point now is that whatever "partnership" we forge won't be entirely comfortable; it won't be entirely equal; it won't be completely free of fear or anxiety. This partnership will take place against a backdrop of institutional expectations on your side and competing concerns on mine. It will be tentative; the trust we both hope for will be contaminated by my skepticism about the profiteering of big pharmaceutical companies and the hidden agendas at work in medical research and perhaps your impatience with repetition or the constant need to explain the obvious.

Also, maybe on your part, the exchange will be fogged by a crowded schedule and what must be a chronic, pressing awareness that more urgent cases are waiting. Still, I need your advice and care. I know many people conserve energy in crisis or uncertainty by simply consigning them-selves to the care of experts, asking no questions, and just hoping you'll "fix it." But I'm not one of them. I don't just want to be told what to do. I want advice, guidance, encouragement, information, direction, and even the benefit of your intuition and best guesses, which I know you may be hesitant to share in a profession that prides itself on practicing "evidence-based medicine."

The notion of "evidence-based medicine" sounds reassuring, but it sometimes begs the question of what the "evidence" actually is. Is my experience evidence? Is yours—even with quirky, unusual cases? How much evi-dence do I need to convince you that eliminating gluten actually helps me, or that nitrates or chlorine may be fac-tors affecting my health? How do you gather and measure evidence of subtle psychosomatic factors in an ongoing stomach disorder? How much may my practice of prayer count as a factor in my healing? Even though you've seen people with my condition before, you haven't seen peo-ple who cope with it as I do or people who have thought about it as I have. So I'm assuming that as I learn from you (and I expect to, because good doctors are always teachers), you may learn from me.

I remember the moment in the film *Awakenings* (1990) when the patient Leonard, beautifully played by

Robert De Niro, realizes that the experimental medicine he's receiving isn't working and he's slipping back into the catatonic state from which he's been temporarily "awakened." Throughout severe seizures, he insists the doctor grab the camera, record what he can, and "Learn! Learn!" It's a beautiful reminder that as I open myself to your help and healing, I also offer you a chance to learn. I want to know whatever may be helpful about what you know. Perhaps that should go both ways.

So, to help us foster a more satisfying partnership, here are some things I'd like you to know that I know or believe. I hope you may consider them as you partner with me in the healing work we both must do.

1. I know there are things you haven't been trained to ask about—or have been trained not to ask about. What you're not asking may limit your ability to help me. I may know things that are more useful than you think. Opening a little more space and time in our conversation (say, around two minutes) for me to say what I believe is true from my own experience and understanding of my condition—what seems to work and what doesn't, what I've read or heard and found convincing, what kinds of "complementary" or "alternative" approaches I have come to trust, how I make my

food choices—may expand your own repertoire of questions and curiosities, and will enrich our conversation about how I may heal. I know it's up to me to decide about what you recommend, and I know those decisions will depend partly on things I know about myself that are not always measurable or even evidence-based in the standard sense, but they matter to me nevertheless.

2. I know that some stressors complicate my condition. I know how my body reacts to conflict with coworkers—and how much of my energy goes into avoiding conflict. I know my blood pressure rises when a supervisor micromanages my projects. I know I get headaches when I take on too much work, and still, "cutting back" often seems neither practical nor possible. I know financial worries affect every aspect of my life. I know the fluctuations in my sleep patterns and my eating patterns (and what may be problematic about them). I also know what helps me take care of myself and what drives me into self-neglect.

3. I know what I've read on the internet about my condition—and before you roll your eyes because every patient you see has read something on the

internet, I know enough to filter out the fad diets and promo ads and to look at WebMD and the Mayo Clinic. I also look at sites and sources that offer insights from "alternative," "complementary," and "integrative" medicine. I may have had more time to research and compare those kinds of sources than you have, given what I know about your demanding schedule. I know some are better than others. I know some offer insights and case studies that are woefully underreported because they come from careful, often courageous, practitioners who have parted company with the big pharmaceutical companies and the American Medical Association (AMA)—a costly decision, and not one I'm suggesting you should make. I know when I'm willing to try what doesn't make rational sense but might help for reasons I don't yet understand. I don't believe conventional chemical and surgery-dominated medicine is always superior to the more mysterious, less empirical modalities of other healing traditions.

4. I know most medical schools don't focus on nutrition, and that food isn't likely a factor in your prescriptions beyond the most general way: eat healthily; avoid too much sugar, salt, caffeine,

and alcohol; get more exercise and sleep. I know there's much more to say about food (and the food system we inhabit) than that, and I believe more of that conversation could be beneficial for both of us. I know there are fine books and documentaries about food as medicine out there along with all the diet hype, and that fine-tuning food practices needs to be part of my health plan.

5. I know that pharmaceutical companies offer you enticing incentives to prescribe their particular drugs, even "off-label," and to use brand names to develop brand loyalty. I know we inhabit food, drug, and "health" industries that are massive, market driven, riddled with conflicts of interest, and disinclined to support research that doesn't promise substantial profit. I know you're not gullible enough to believe the pitch of every pharm rep who brings samples to your office, but I also know a barrage of incentives may be hard to resist, and unbiased information hard to come by, so what you prescribe may sometimes be a time-saving default option.

6. I know that my spirituality and faith inform my approach to illness, and I know your office isn't

necessarily the place to talk about that, but it may be a place to acknowledge it. Making room for a faith factor could open a space in the conversation for mystery, possibility, and surprise.

You know far more than I do about the wide range of organic problems and processes covered in medical school courses. And you know far more than I do about what patients are unlikely to know, what they tend to miss, what they believe too readily, what remedies help common conditions, and what's happening at the cutting edge of cancer treatment, prenatal care, public health provision, and micro-surgery. I don't question your competence and expertise in your field; I'm very grateful for the ways I benefit from them. I also know I will benefit most if we both recognize we're in it together—partnering in finding out what might work this time because it's not last time—because "everyone is a special case."

I'd like a long relationship with you. I think doctors and patients work best together if they know one another. These days, I count on you to see to many "ordinary" medical needs—flu vaccines, routine blood tests, possible ways to address deepening fatigue, information about bone density. When the time comes, I'd like to know I have a doctor I can trust to see me through the harder things—injury, serious illness, dying. Like many, I've read Paul Kalanithi's *When Breath Becomes Air*, a moving account of a young neurosurgeon who reflects on his condition as both doctor and patient as he is dying:

> I feared I was losing sight of the singular importance of human relationships, not between patients and their families but between doctor and patient. Technical excellence was not enough. As a resident, my highest ideal was not saving lives—everyone dies eventually—but guiding a patient or family to an understanding of death or illness. When a patient comes in with a fatal head bleed, that first conversation with a neurosurgeon may forever color how the family remembers the death . . . When there's no place for the scalpel, words are the surgeon's only tool.

Words are a valuable tool. We both have access to many of them. I'm grateful for whatever authenticity, generous curiosity, humility, and grace we can bring to the work of healing and maintaining health. Beneath the roles of doctor and patient, I trust we can meet one another as human beings who are learning to be human together until, inevitably, death comes. And then we find out what's next.

My Two Minutes: Do you have a good story about partnering with a patient in some way that went beyond good "bedside manner?" What made that work more collaborative"?

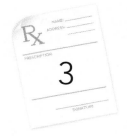

ON BEING A
SPECIAL CASE

Everyone is a special case.

—ALBERT CAMUS

MY HISTORY OF PAIN has been far less arduous than what many others have had to endure, but it has offered me valuable learning moments. Migraines, broken bones, nephritis, pinched discs, ulcers, smashed fingers, pulled muscles, and one bout of clinical depression have given me sufficient occasion to muse about pain and suffering. Inclining to theological questions—a habit acquired from a childhood spent with devout missionary parents—I've asked myself how personal suffering might serve divine purposes, how it might contribute to spiritual growth, how it might deepen my capacity for compassion.

On occasion, suffering has also made me cranky, disheartened, withdrawn, self-pitying, or anxious. Other people's suffering remains a disturbing mystery that sometimes makes it very hard to watch the news. Beyond donating to Doctors Without Borders, or Partners in Health, or voting for improvements in health care, it often seems nearly impossible for ordinary people like me to help alleviate it.

I'm aware, especially in a pandemic that is spreading even as I write this, of how suffering takes place in political and family systems. I am privileged to have the resources I need to deal with pain. I've lain in darkened rooms practicing techniques for riding waves of pain or diving into them, breathing through the throbbing, observing the pain and detaching, listening to music someone thoughtfully provided, reciting scraps of poetry like mantras to get through the worst of it. I'm aware of how many don't have access to those darkened rooms. I've sat with other people, whose pain I can barely imagine, and learned from them how personal a challenge pain is. No two cases of shingles, or bee stings, or flu, or congestive heart failure are the same.

I'm not a textbook case. No one is. None of us quite "fits the profile." My body is a map of my physical and emotional history. My pain has its own geography; it lodges in joints, muscles, nerve paths, and organs for reasons worth knowing, though not always knowable. I know that when I'm emotionally overwrought, I feel it in my stomach. When I'm frustrated or stressed by unresolved conflicts, my neck hurts. My body remembers things my mind has forgotten.

You, as a doctor, may give me a sound physiological explanation for my shoulder pain, or nausea, or recurrent ache in the left side, but it may be that the "why" question also opens paths of reflection on more than physiological facts and can lead into territory that is shadowy and intimate and thick with undergrowth and uncertainties. For me to understand fully why I carry pain the way I do may require more curiosity and patience than you're trained, or even allowed, to have. You might rightly refer me to a good therapist, or spiritual director, or old friend for that conversation. But just play with this: What might happen if you were to follow me a little way down that path and see what we both could learn? Because though I'm not a textbook case, my case might make a good teaching tale.

Pain is hard to articulate. It certainly can't be adequately described on a "scale of one to ten." My pain chooses its own moments and travels its own pathways. My stomachaches occur rather predictably in response to particular kinds of stress—e.g., being around other people's anger or fear of missing a deadline. My headaches travel down one side of my head, behind my eye, and into my neck. Those headaches develop in stages: early on, they beat out a rhythm, later they fill the space inside my skull and spill out into the air I breathe. As I try to describe them, my language grows more fanciful. Sometimes the pain flickers; other times it oozes or pounds or thickens. It radiates, or penetrates, or suffuses.

I once worked with a biofeedback practitioner who encouraged movement toward figurative language with questions like these: *What color is your headache? How big is it? What shape is it? Can you move it? Where can you send it?* I remember, as I considered that last one, thinking about the incident in the Gospel of Matthew where Jesus sends demons into a hapless herd of pigs and they dive over a cliff. As no herd of pigs was handy for me at the time, and I still would have hesitated to disturb their peace, I abandoned that image. However, on one notable occasion, I did "send" the headache away successfully. The headaches come less frequently now. The work I've done with them and other kinds of pain have enabled me to bring more imagination to conversations about pain. Finding the "right" word or image can release or relax the body's defensive grip and restore a healing flow of energy in ways that are not often described in textbooks. I could use your help in finding those "right" words.

I share this bit of history to invite you to think with me about how to address my pain as a personal matter that a numerical rating system cannot measure.

Maybe poetry will help. Here's an exquisite poem titled "Stranded" about post-surgery pain by Karen Fiser, a woman who has lived for years with more pain than I have ever had to face. It has helped me remember both the surprising uniqueness and the multidimensionality of physical suffering:

> Gasping at the bed's edge
> you cling to the sour pillow
> of sand, flounder through
> the briny sheets, held
> out of your damaged body's
> element. You keep struggling
> in the shallows for the right
> kind of breath. Something
> you can never fathom
> drove you here. Think hard,
> so hard it hurts.
> Call out all you want.
> You can't get back to the rest
> of your life, to finish it.

I hope this poem will lead you to others. I hope it inspires you to reflect on patients' pain in new ways—how waking into pain is an experience of bewilderment, shock, and loss, as if tossed up on a beach, alone and gasping. I remember learning to body surf, failing, flailing, choking on salty water, scraping my skin on sand. There is a moment of feeling safe; then another wave comes and you "struggle in the shallows," tantalizingly near shore and respite but still tugged downward and outward.

People in pain often speak of waves, of being pulled under, of drowning. I remember the pain of childbirth that way; the trick was to ride the waves. Sometimes, you couldn't. You went under. You came up gasping. In my case, there were three happy outcomes. Even so, I couldn't get back to the rest of my life, any more than the speaker in this poem, because "back" isn't where you go. I have come to understand how not only childbirth, but any significant experience of pain, leaves you changed. You carry it in your consciousness. It leaves its mark on the psyche and in the cells.

Poets have taught me much about pain and helped me explore my own. In another of her poems, Fiser speaks about how surgery, hospitalization, and chronic pain change everything—ambient sound, color, memory—and how pain continues to bewilder. *Bewilder* is a word I've paused over often—it's not the first one people associate with pain, but it's an important one. Pain can make you wild—reduce you to the hypervigilance of animals who know they are being pursued. It makes you self-aware in new ways—of your raw sentience and your mortality.

When I talk with you about pain, I'd like you to know it's interesting when it's not overwhelming. Its peculiarities, subtle shifts, and changes; the way sound or odors affect it; or the steady, intelligent touch of a hand or guided meditations—all are valuable information to me—especially the way pain evokes images. How I imagine my pain matters.

I remember seeing an exhibit of headache art in Cambridge, Massachusetts, that featured visual images drawn or painted by people who suffered from migraines or similar syndromes. It was a wild, colorful, disturbing array that featured various waves and rays, or sharp objects entering the eye, or flames along jawbones and temples, or spiky circles like crowns of thorns. There were screws and hammers and picks and spikes, as well as rather beautiful wavy lines where a face used to be. I once drew a picture of myself with a migraine. In it, I was encased in a black cocoon with a halo of bright spikes around my head. It made me realize that part of the experience of migraine for me was one of isolation, enclosure, and suffocating insularity. Yet a cocoon is also an image of something temporary—a second skin that will disintegrate on its own. It promises restoration and emergence. It comes with a reassurance that I'm not going to die, no matter how much the body throbs and threatens. In migraine art, colors matter, size matters, shapes matter. Even the most conventional images offer encoded information.

Pain, in other words, can activate the imagination. It occurs where the body, with its web of nerves and myriad sensations, intersects with mind and spirit. It is malleable and surprising. Language and images can actually help to dispel pain or at least redirect it. At least I've found that to be true. I've come to believe all pain and suffering have a psychosomatic dimension, that we hold and locate pain in our bodies in idiosyncratic and sometimes rather creative ways, though I imagine most of us don't consciously choose those ways.

Even if you don't think about pain quite as fancifully, I need you to know that I do. Not because I expect you to be a dream analyst, or therapist, or even a reader of poetry (though I recommend it), but because images offer information, and how I experience and express pain could help fine-tune diagnosis and treatment.

To really consider that information might require an extra measure of interest and willingness on your part. Discussing how I think about my pain might take the whole extra two minutes my medical educator friend asked her med students to imagine. Those could be two minutes well spent.

If you take two minutes with me, and two more minutes with another patient, you may find yourself on a learning curve about varieties of painful experience, about the sometimes-magical power of words and images, and about how much healing can happen even when pain continues. One poet who suffers intense migraines, Linda Pastan, imagines herself crouching "on the / tilting floor of / consciousness," a visual that names the vertiginous feeling that can come during a severe headache with a certain precision, altering one's sense of place or location in space. Alexandre Arnau, another migraine sufferer, writes of

a torn bit
of light
beating ceaseless
hidden codes
behind my
frail bleeding
eyes.

I'm intrigued in those lines by how "codes" suggests meaning in suffering that has to be broken open or discovered.

A third poet, Katherine Larson, describes migraine as a "dark anchor" lodged behind the eyes. And another, Cathy Song, recounts her exploration of pain with the precision of a scientific observer:

> When I touch my eyelids,
> my hands react as if
> I had just touched something
> hot enough to burn.
> My skin, aspirin colored,
> tingles with migraine.

I want you, to whom I turn for help in healing, to know this: pain teaches me; and while I want relief, I don't always want it at the cost of understanding. I value information, whether it comes from the "wise woman within," or from websites that cite recent studies, or from TED talks by scientists, or simply from people I meet whose pain is similar to mine. I don't want to miss what I might learn from suffering. So I'd value an extra minute of instruction from you, perhaps with a scribbled diagram, about physiological processes, or about how a drug works, or how particular foods might help or hurt.

I'd like your help not only as a health care provider, but also as an educator, to explore my pathologies so I can decide what to do about them. Like teaching and learning, healing seems to involve an exchange that's personal and relational. Not everyone wants or needs to learn the same lessons about illness or pain.

What I need to know and what I want to know have much to do with what I'm ready to know. I realize I protect myself from too much information when it threatens to become overwhelming, or confusing, or fatiguing to process. I may want to explore how meditation and slow, deep breathing can help, but not take a full course of instruction in prana yoga. I may be willing to focus on recognizing and reducing daily stress, but not willing to change my job or social habits since I may still be getting enough satisfaction from them to counterbalance the stress. I may need help sorting those out and assessing the tradeoffs. A few timely questions from you could help me do that, especially as you are someone who knows my medical history. Others have another piece of the picture. They know about my mood swings, my values, and my habits.

No one knows those things more than the people I live among and love. How I heal depends, in part, on family, friends, conversation, food, recreation, and recognition. Knowing and being known create the context in which I work out my health and healing. I know that my suffering, when it comes, affects those around me. My husband has learned all my signs of pain and fatigue. The suffering taps the delicate floating mobile of family life and shifts our roles and relationships into reeling, tipping arcs.

Sometimes I want to talk about it. Sometimes I don't. As I work out my needs, some of my family back away; others move in closer. Some pick up my duties while others bring vegetable bouillon and keep the phone away. They also teach me what I need. They experiment to see what helps, and we all learn in the process what "help" means. I learn I need touch and quiet and that it helps me to have someone just reading, or breathing, or resting nearby. I know others' prayers and good wishes do matter, sometimes in ways I can feel but barely fathom. I know my role in my family system will shape my decisions about how to handle my own suffering, and sometimes that role needs to be reexamined and revised.

However limited your time is, I'd like you to remember and acknowledge that my story isn't the same as others' stories. I know from pregnant women, and from people undergoing chemo, and from people with back pain, allergies, or insomnia, that disclosing those conditions often elicits a description of what the doctor typically sees. Others who have suffered similar conditions give an oddly enthusiastic "Me too!" They've "been through this." They have advice and sympathy to offer. Some irritatingly substitute the former for the latter. Some are remarkably empathetic. Most respond with compassion. But they haven't traveled my path. Every journey digresses into new territory because every body has its own geography. We may not be islands, but we do make solo voyages into what Susan Sontag called "the kingdom of the sick."

That voyage of relief from physical suffering is not the only thing I seek. At the risk of violating a dearly held standard of professional detachment, I would be so bold as to suggest that what I need—and what I believe every patient needs in some measure—is a medical professional's intelligent imagination, loving kindness, and open-hearted curiosity that asks *who* as well as *what* they may find in the shivering body perched partly clad on the exam table.

When I come to see you, it is with the hope that our encounter can offer us both something broaching a sacred moment. That may seem not only an excessive, but perhaps even an inappropriate, expectation. Still, I believe real healing requires an environment of sincerity and interest rooted in a deep sense that we are in it together—vulnerable, and mortal, and resilient. Something we might boldly call love can be exchanged with complete professional respect when we find ourselves in a conversation that might, in two extra minutes, take us beyond problems needing fixing into a place of mystery where simple certainties give way to humble amazement at what may be possible.

My Two Minutes: How do you maintain your curiosity about each case? How do you bring a "beginner's mind" to each encounter?

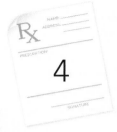

WORDS MATTER

Words can strengthen the weak, words can reju-
venate the meek—words can breathe life into the
dead . . . words can encourage the hearts of the
desperate—words can alleviate the anguish of
humanity, words can sow the seeds of serenity.
—ABHIJIT NASKAR, *TIME TO SAVE MEDICINE*

Words, after speech, reach
Into the silence.

—T. S. ELIOT

WORDS MATTER TO ME. How you put things makes a
difference: how accessible your language is; how careful
you are to define, or explain, or illustrate what might be
unfamiliar; how carefully you listen to my words and care

about the way I account for my experience. I'm aware that in any urban practice these days, there are likely patients from multiple language groups; medical translators aren't hard up for jobs. However, even when you talk with me or any other English-speaking patient who is not a physician, you're translating.

You have acquired a specialized vocabulary—Latin names for body parts, long compound words with Greek roots, terms from pharmacology and biochemistry—of which most of us have limited understanding. You need those terms, and we need you to know them, for the way they link you to a whole history of scientific systems. "Learning medicine," Daniel Kahneman wrote, "consists in part of learning the language of medicine. A deeper understanding of judgments and choices also requires a richer vocabulary than is available in everyday language."

I've done translations, though not in your field. I know it's exacting, but not exact. It may be simple to say *inflammation of the heart* instead of *myocarditis*, or *enlarged liver* instead of *hepatomegaly*, but it is a little more difficult to explain how a beta blocker works or what an antihyperlipidemic agent is. Those require a little basic physiology and organic chemistry. Or some homely images. I know it's hard to simplify without dumbing down, but know from my own experience as an educated, but anxious, patient that it's important to do the former and avoid the latter. They're different. The public suffers from dumbed-down reporting on complicated matters like climate change, military actions, and the economy. We need skillful, public-minded experts to help us grasp the complexities so we can respond appropriately. That takes reflection and patience and discernment about how to condense, what to omit, and where to define. I like physicist Richard Feynman's response to a journalist who asked him to describe what he'd won the Nobel Prize for in three minutes. He said if he could explain it in three minutes, it wouldn't be worth a Nobel Prize. Too many experts, under the sudden pressure of microphone and camera, or simply the time pressures of a work day, resort to sound bites that oversimplify. But it's possible to simplify without *over*simplifying. Patients like me need good popularizers more than ever as the distance between general and specialized knowledge grows. Democracy and public safety and health require that we all be carefully informed about how drugs work, what may be their side effects, how they are produced, who controls their cost, how insurance systems work to patients' advantage, and how we can find out when some of them put stockholders' interests over patients'. Aurora Levins Morales, writing about the culture and politics of medicine, makes an eloquent plea on behalf of all of us who need to know more about medicine to make decisions that are more informed:

> To do exciting, empowering research and leave it in academic journals and university libraries is like manufacturing unaffordable medicines for deadly diseases. We need to share our work in ways that people can assimilate, not in the private languages and forms of scholars . . . Those who are hungriest for what we dig up don't read scholarly journals and shouldn't have to.

This is a heartening plea for the public interest and a reminder that you medical folk are also educators. It's part of your job. I believe that to communicate well—to foster understanding that includes empathy, imagination, and intuition—we all must hear and speak words with some awareness of how and what they "trigger," the cultural and personal associations they may awaken, how they may be "loaded," and how, at times, they can have a "sacramental" effect that imparts blessing, energy, hope, or peace. This obligation seems especially incumbent upon professionals who have information and perspectives the rest of us need.

Sometimes a single word will awaken an insight neither you nor I could have anticipated. Sometimes a word or phrase will open my heart. Sometimes it will make me defensive.

And on that subject, a language matter that may seem trivial to you is how we address each other. I like informality; I like being addressed by my first name. When it doesn't go both ways, it's disconcerting. We're both adults. We both, as it happens, have graduate degrees. Both of us carry the title "Dr." in our professional lives. Given also that I'm nearly twice your age at this point, there's something unsettling in expecting that I use your title when you don't use mine. Yes, you're the one wearing the white coat and it's your workplace, but maybe we could address each other in a way that enables us both to find a good balance between formality and familiarity as we negotiate a conversation that may have a fair number of sticky wickets. Or potholes. Or sand traps. Or rocky stretches. Maybe as we go, we can find amusing moments and simple pleasures in being human together, if only with an inventive turn of phrase or a pun.

Happily, the importance of language in medicine has been brought to public attention in new ways over the past several decades. Most of us are now aware that "disability" is preferable to "handicap" and "person with diabetes" is preferable to "diabetic." Most of us are aware of how "othering" works, how ways of naming illnesses and

45

people with those illnesses, and assigning people to fixed categories make the uniqueness of individuals less visible. On the other hand, the names of particular disorders, diseases, and syndromes—the autism spectrum, ADD, ADHD, various autoimmune diseases—have come into common use, enabling us all to recognize with greater specificity, and therefore greater understanding and compassion, what persons who live with those conditions may be experiencing.

I'd like to highlight five ways words have come to matter to me in our clinical conversations. The first is your use, and mine, of explanatory metaphors or similes. You're handy with a simile. Encouraging me to care for my teeth "as I would for my most precious jewels," though I don't really own precious jewels, has helped me floss and brush even when I'm tired and tempted to wait until morning. And suggesting that the fluctuation of pain may follow musical patterns has allowed me a certain helpful, interested distance on the pain when it comes. Maybe you have read Anatole Broyard's book *Intoxicated by My Illness*, with its fascinating reflections on metaphors in medicine. I find myself nodding emphatically when he says, for instance:

> Metaphors may be as necessary to illness as they
> are to literature, as comforting to the patient as

his own bathrobe and slippers. At the very least, they are a relief from medical terminology . . . Perhaps only metaphor can express the bafflement, the panic combined with beatitude, of the threatened person.

I appreciate that acknowledgment; I think metaphors are not only useful, but inevitable. However, some of them, as I'll reflect on in the next chapter, are unhelpful and obstructive. The most common metaphors I'm aware of in American medicine are those that come from military language (*fighting disease*, *being a trooper*, *soldiering on*, *battling cancer*, *an arsenal of drugs*, *bombarding a site with antibiotics*, *aggressive treatment*, *armies of white blood cells*, etc.). They deserve their own discussion. Suffice it to say they're problematic because of the mindset they create, the strategies they invoke, and the way they compete with practices aimed at cultivating deep inner peace.

Other common metaphors come from sports (*staying in the game*, *riding the wave*, *the Hail Mary pass*, *how you change strategies in the seventh inning*, *slam dunk*, etc.). I can see how these might energize sports fans. Some of them even energize me. Learning to "ride the wave" of pain helped me through childbirth; and later through long, throbbing headaches; and then while waiting for a gastric ulcer to heal. Sports metaphors, unlike military ones, at least call on experiences that are more accessible. It might be useful to ask me and other patients what sports we've played to choose the most meaningful metaphors for the occasion. Tennis, basketball, bodysurfing, and skating images evoke memories much more effectively for me than golf, weight lifting, or football.

I think of how many moments in a tennis match are spent waiting in readiness to see what happens—e.g., from which angle the serve comes, and with what force. That seems like a kind of alert attentiveness training that's applicable to a treatment whose effects must be closely observed. Or how the "full court press" in basketball might help clarify the need for aggressive treatments. Or how bodysurfing on Southern California beaches, being carried in by a wave to where my belly meets the sand, feeling vulnerable and exhilarated as I surrender to a force of nature, taught me to say yes to something both fearful and challenging, and find joy in it. Riding waves of pain, riding out the effects of prolonged treatment, those memories help me.

Other common metaphors come from the world of manufacturing and machines. Those can help clarify process (for instance, pointing out the way the digestive system gets "clogged" like plumbing), but I don't like the way they reduce the intricate, complex, organic, body-mind-spirit to an object with replaceable parts. It's easiest to fall into this kind of language regarding surgery—to presume that ovaries, or appendices, or even lungs or hearts are dispensable or replaceable parts. There's no room in that language to acknowledge that surgery often changes people's hormonal balances, or immune responses, or general resilience, or that it may have lasting psychological effects.

You might enjoy an essay by Dr. Vyjeyanthi S. Periyakoil that distinguishes two ways metaphors can be useful in medicine. One is to "introduce unfamiliar material" to patients who need to know, say, why chemotherapy makes them lose their hair or what the difference is between two types of diabetes, or how autoimmune diseases work. The other is to "break preexisting mind-sets," deconstructing common assumptions to help patients think more complexly or accurately about their conditions and their choices. I'm grateful for the imagination and ingenuity you, or any doctor, brings to making complicated things comprehensible. With a little imagination on both sides, maybe we can navigate the rough waters of disease. Or run the obstacle course. Or pick our way across the minefield. Or slash through the thicket. Or find a quiet cave and wait out the storm.

Words matter in other ways when we talk about illness, injury, or treatment. The conversation seems most helpful to me when we discuss *my* experience of *my* condition, as well as general information about what the symptoms indicate and what is likely to be appropriate standard treatment. I appreciate getting a chance to explain how I respond to pain, or talk about what my treatment plan may require of the people I live with, or about anxieties that may be irrational, but are a very real part of the problem to be addressed.

I'm grateful for words of comfort while being given information or instruction. I'm grateful for a touch of appropriate humor here and there—an aside about how to capitalize on a chic eye patch or how a crutch or sling can start conversations with sympathetic strangers. I'm grateful for plain language that avoids not only abstruse medical jargon but also clichés from the corporate world—words like "deliverables" or "value added" or "managing expectations" or being "proactive." Trendy language like that can be generation-specific, tiresomely or flatly optimistic rather than informative and hopeful, and suggest that the very human, intimate, fleshly, nuanced, spiritually significant matter of disease can be reduced to cost-benefit analyses, actuarial calculations, and prescriptive "bottom lines."

It also seems especially important to develop rich, compassionate, open-ended ways of talking about death and dying, even if I'm not there yet. I won't generalize, but I've known many doctors who will go to some lengths to avoid any conversation about death that involves more than delivering the bad news of a terminal prognosis. I need you not to be one of them. On medical reticence about dying, Sunita Puri in *That Good Night: Life and Medicine in the Eleventh Hour,* points out sharply, "Lacking the language to discuss mortality is the ultimate way of erasing it." I don't know if anyone has ever been sued for malpractice because of an inability to acknowledge what was happening when death approached, but perhaps some should have been. I have witnessed reticence of this kind that amounted to withholding life-support.

My work as a hospice volunteer has led me to think about and experiment with words regarding death in conversation with patients (some religious, some decidedly not) who seem to want and need them. For some, silence is the most appropriate gift to bring to the bedside during the final days or hours. But many want to talk about death—what we can know about what it's like, what I've learned about death from being with others as they died, what can we learn from the many reported instances of "near-death experiences." Others appreciate poems or readings from sacred texts. While I've developed my own repertoire of favorites, I have learned that even poems I find a little too "Hallmark" can sometimes touch a chord for people, so it seems a good time to lay my literary judgments aside and read aloud whatever offers comfort. (When my time comes, though, if you're anywhere nearby, bear in mind that a life of teaching literature has given me opinions, so indulge them, please!) A dear friend of mine, a highly skilled singer who instructed many world-class opera singers, recommended that her students make a playlist of things they'd like to hear in their final days if they were no longer able to voice their preferences. She herself put her own list to use during the sad, gracious season of her own death. I mention that here because the same could be done with poems or passages. Words of comfort come from a wide variety of sources, such as Aeschylus's reference to wisdom that comes to us "in our own despair, against our will" by "the awful grace of God"; and the final lines of Jane Kenyon's exquisite poem, "Let Evening Come": "Let it come, as it will, and don't / be afraid. God will not leave us comfortless, so / Let evening come."

Comfort is a word we use freely and often in hospice. It seems, for evident reasons, to receive less emphasis in medical training, though good doctors and their students do talk about it. And though you aren't the first person I'd turn to for comfort while in distress—I have a husband and family folk and friends and priests who can offer that—you might be the one I'd most need it from in a moment of confronting a life-changing diagnosis or death's unexpected imminence. And because you might be that person, I hope you consider comfort as one of the basic clinical skills you're responsible for developing.

Comfort doesn't, I hasten to clarify, consist of minimizing or trivializing or diminishing the weight, cost, or pain of what a patient is undergoing. I think of when I've heard some doctors toss off a word like "just," for instance. If the alarming new blotch that has spread suddenly on my arm is "just" a blood blister, I'm glad to know that, but the sentence without the "just" can reassure me that it's not melanoma without dismissing my initial concerns as silly ignorance or hypochondria. Even though "just" is often meant to restore a reassuring perspective, it can feel gratingly condescending. Real comfort begins in full, empathetic acknowledgment of the scope of sorrow or anxiety, and enters into a moment of need with simplicity and kindness.

In Abraham Verghese's beautiful novel about coming of age into a life in medicine, *Cutting for Stone*, the narrator recalls a learning moment with his physician father: "'Tell us please, what treatment in an emergency is administered by ear?'" the father asks. "I met his gaze and I did not blink. 'Words of comfort,' I said to my father." Sometimes they're the only medicine available, and you may be the only one to provide it. I hope you have some. Even simple ones are remarkably helpful: "This pain will lessen." "Your body knows how to do what it needs to do." "There are a lot of people ready to help you." I hope you consider what gives you comfort in hard times; you, who witness other people's anguish or anxiety regularly, must sometimes lie awake at night laden with those sorrows and your own. I wonder what helps you. I hope you find ways to share that help in a spirit that moves you beyond the role of a trained practitioner to that of a fellow traveler who may be able to see a little further down a path we're both on.

The reflection below on the comfort of words is from a woman whose native language group has had to survive against great odds. Joyce Sequichie Hifler restores words to their rightful place among instruments of healing and human flourishing:

> There is power in a word, whether we read it, speak it or hear it. And we command and are commanded by the word. We scatter, we call forth, and we comfort. Words are tools, weapons,

both good and bad medicine. . . . The word, or *ka ne tsv* in Cherokee, is power to help heal, or make sick people sicker by negative talk around them. The word gives confidence when it builds rather than destroys. . . . Until we listen to our own voices and how we talk, we would never guess how we use our words.

As we continue to learn how to engage in life-giving conversation, I hope we can "listen to our own voices" and make "good medicine" of the words we exchange.

My Two Minutes: Are there particular words that have become "watchwords" for you in your work? Sentences that you come back to? Mantras, prayers, sayings that help you stay centered and attentive?

A Quieter Way

In Beyond AIDS: A Journey into Healing, George Melton is clear in defining his own stance as markedly different from that of the patient who is a "fighter." He remarks, "I knew my health would not come as a result of fighting my illness, but rather as a by-product of seeking my connection to the power within me."

—ANNE HUNSAKER HAWKINS, *RECONSTRUCTING ILLNESS: STUDIES IN PATHOGRAPHY*

I DON'T LIKE AGGRESSION. I don't like to fight. I don't like watching battle scenes in movies or other spectacles of violence that have become almost tediously normal. I don't even like verbal arguments; they leave me unsettled and unsatisfied. I don't think war is ever "the answer" nor violence a sensible way to "keep peace." And I think competitiveness is an oversung "virtue." Therefore, when I'm sick, I don't want to fight.

I know people who do. I heard many a mutual friend say admiringly of a colleague dying of cancer, "She's a fighter." She was. And she did die, but not without pursuing every promising means (some very distasteful and painful, and some odd and, I thought, unpromising) to stay alive and watch her kids grow. I've witnessed gentle, gracious people's long struggles with sickle cell anemia, or Gaucher disease, or multiple sclerosis (MS) in which words like *fighting*, *combating*, *resisting*, *battling*, *tactics*, and an *arsenal* of drugs occurred with remarkable frequency. These people submitted to aggressive treatment. They took orders. And they sustained hard hits with fortitude I admire.

But war metaphors have shaped medicine in ways I find disturbing and repellant. There's a lot of war going on around the planet, much of it in city streets where children are maimed by "smart bombs" and lone survivors of large families find shelter in rubble. It's ugly. It's horrifying. Individual losses and injuries are "collateral damage." Ecosystems and infrastructures are destroyed. And yet, the military metaphors persist. We keep hearing about the "wars" supposedly being waged on cancer, drugs, poverty.

In "The Military Metaphors of Modern Medicine," Abraham Fuks reminds clinical practitioners like you, whose professional language may be laced with the rhetoric of warfare:

> Medical discourse is replete with the language of war and such phrases as "the war on cancer," "magic bullets," "silver bullets," "the therapeutic armamentarium," "agents of disease," "the body's defences," and "doctor's orders" are deeply engrained in our medical rhetoric. The mindset engendered by this discourse of war renders the patient as a battlefield upon which the doctor-combatant defeats the arch-enemy, disease.

Imagining my body as a battleground doesn't give me the inner peace I need to make my way along the hard stretches on the path toward healing. Fighting, one of the most common metaphors you seem to reach for when you want to encourage the ill and infirm, doesn't work for me.

I'd rather negotiate. Whether I'm doing so with people, or with cells and tissues, or with my inner critic, or any of the other furtive folk who lurk in the back rooms of my psyche, I'd much rather seek nonviolent solutions to problems than take aggressive measures that leave unaccounted wreckage in their wake. Let's look at alternatives to "winning and losing"—adapting, accommodating, mitigating, exploring. We can sideline the language of the military campaign. Once we start sending in warships and staging drone attacks, we're unlikely to put much energy into imagining a middle way or understanding those we've identified as the enemy. But when I'm facing a health threat (and this includes the public health threats that we're all facing, such as pesticides and other pollutants, carcinogens, stronger strains of known viruses, zoonotic diseases entering human populations, etc.) I want some clear, reasonable alternatives to "fighting."

I want you to talk with me about ways to care for my general health. I want to understand my immune system and give it all the help I can. I'd like to take a moment here and there with an educated caregiver to review what my liver needs, what may enable deeper rest, and how to recognize what foods, activities, and environments are life-giving and healthy with more specificity. I'd like help navigating the wilderness of pharmaceutical ads, health claims on cereal boxes, and health warnings without the mounting anxiety, which, itself, so quickly affects sleep, digestion, and peace of mind.

If I have to live with an illness for any length of time, I want you to help me reimagine my life in new terms and help me adopt them. If I can't play tennis any more, will my shoulder tolerate pickleball? If I do better when I avoid noisy restaurants or spicy food, maybe I need encouragement to seek out other pleasures altogether, such as enjoying my friends on walks or over game boards. Taking account of my body's new vulnerabilities as I walk through my own illnesses or witness others' changes my standards for and expectations of myself. As I age, even if I "age well," I know I have to keep making small accommodations.

Friends who have suffered injury or encroaching disabilities like MS, or arthritis, or Parkinson's have had to reorganize not only their routines, but also their hopes and ambitions. They've had to adapt to relative immobility. They've had to keep things on lower shelves or use mechanical devices for picking things up off the floor. They've had to familiarize themselves with which sidewalk routes are navigable by wheelchair. They've had to attach raised toilet seats or buy hats and scarves to get through months of hair loss.

Adaptation isn't the same as capitulation. I think of the poignant question Dhruv Khullar raised in another piece about military metaphors in medicine when he asks about a patient who died after a fruitless "fight": "Did she, on some level, feel she lost the battle because she didn't fight hard enough? Might she have suffered less at the end if she hadn't felt compelled to try one more drug, determined to soldier on?"

"People telling you to 'keep fighting' when you're feeling weak or having a low day makes you feel as though you're doing something wrong or even worse, being cowardly," one breast cancer survivor writes. I know some people need that encouragement. But those who choose to find a quieter way, who choose the language of self-nurturing, who see inner peace and whatever wisdom may be available in the experience, sometimes find themselves like pacifists and conscientious objectors who are accused of being cowards by those for whom fighting is not only normative, but also a compulsory test of courage.

Where there is humiliation in "losing," there is dignity in accepting what one can't change while changing the things one can, as people in a twelve-step program are regularly reminded. On what terms each of us finds "strength in what remains" is a personal, lively question that might be addressed at least briefly in conversation with you, as my health care provider, whose calling and curiosities lie in healing. I'd like your help with a range of responses other than fighting.

I'd like help redirecting my energies. My reservoir of available energy may dwindle when I'm ill or in pain, but

I can still choose how to use my waking hours. If, instead of "fighting" I turn inward; focus on slow, deep breathing; meditate, pray; or listen to healing music or guided meditations, I can develop a whole new relationship with my body and the Self who dwells at the center, one that is wiser and more stable than the ego self. If I choose to learn rather than to fight, both that inner teacher and, I hope, one or more sympathetic practitioners who understand their opportunities as teachers, may effect a kind of healing that aggressive interventions can't accomplish.

I'd like help learning to *manage* pain—managing being quite different from *defeating* or *overcoming*. I know from several friends who live with chronic or recurrent pain that, though one of the great benefits of modern medicine is pain relief, this relief often comes at a high price—both in dollars and in side effects like addiction. Pain relievers, as you know, often treat symptoms rather than root causes, postponing deeper healing in favor of immediate respite. And let me say, I'm more than happy to receive respite when I'm in pain. But more than that, I want help with the longer-run project of managing the pain I'm likely to live with—or, if it can be eradicated, finding a deeper, more lasting way to do so than the quick fix.

I'd like help releasing whatever needs to go to clear a way for healing. That might entail your asking very specific questions about what it's time to let go of or prompting questions I need to ask myself: *Am I done with parts of my library? The unfinished projects long stored in the closet? The heavy kitchen appliances I use less and less frequently as I eat more simply? The clutter that might make way for the air and light and openness I need now?* When I'm in a place of illness, or fatigue, or weakness, I think of the various mentors, poets, and spiritual teachers who have reiterated the deceptively simple advice to "let go" when the time comes—even of those things we hold dear and of the people we most cherish and of our own lives when the time comes. It's part of the assignment. Meditating on mortality, and accepting it, can offer healing that can't be received while we're fighting.

All of these—releasing, relearning, managing, letting go—are alternatives to fighting. Fighting precludes these subtler kinds of work and often comes at the expense of peace, or self-understanding, or the spiritual awakening suffering can sometimes offer.

My issues with fighting are not only a matter of personal preference, they are ethical. If a gentler way is possible, I prefer it both in resolving differences and in attending to my body. Aggressive medicine may have its advantages, but the long-term side effects of assaults on disease often seem underestimated and underreported.

Invasive treatments change a person. I know this from watching friends who have gone through aggressive chemotherapy, major surgery, and heavy drug regimens because their doctors (not to mention pharmaceutical ads and fellow sufferers) have urged them to suit up (or disrobe) and enter the war effort. That effort has cost them dearly.

So I'm offering you a friendly challenge. When I have an appointment with you, if you have difficult news to share, avoid the language of warfare. I'd like you to talk with me about the journey I'm taking over this unfamiliar terrain; how to navigate the pitching waves; or how to listen inwardly, quiet my mind, and deepen my acquaintance with my own body. If I have to submit to chemotherapy, or surgery, or any other invasive procedures, I'd like to do even that in ways that emphasize how to strengthen the body's ability to heal itself. I'd like to shore up, deepen, strengthen, reimagine, equip, allow, and care for myself. The thing I don't want to do is fight.

My Two Minutes: How do you cultivate gentleness? What are your own alternatives to fighting?

Noun or Verb

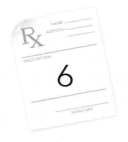

> I know that I am not a category. I am not a thing—
> a noun. I seem to be a verb, an evolutionary
> process.
>
> —R. BUCKMINSTER FULLER

OCCASIONALLY, I STILL SEE someone wearing a T-shirt that reads, "This is what 50 looks like." It was probably a birthday gift. It's a bold thing to wear as it certainly makes passersby take a second glance and presumably consider what they thought 50 looked like while assessing the T-shirt wearer's youthfulness. Anyone who has attended a class reunion has seen, sometimes shockingly, how differently people age, and has had to revise whatever idea of "50" they had beforehand.

As with age, so with ethnicity, class, gender, and regional identities: they're slippery and malleable. I need you to know that when I check boxes on a medical questionnaire, I often wish for a few extra lines to qualify or explain, since I can see that the sketchy information those forms provide is piecemeal and possibly misleading. It's dangerously easy to slide from "Who are you?" to "What are you?"—especially when identity markers are reduced to boxes to be checked. As I'm sure you recognize, to see a person in terms of the category or condition becomes a way of defining them and often forms the basis for prejudgments.

Categories solidify more quickly than ice in a freezer. Convenient descriptors like *white, female, urban, married, professional, Protestant, Democrat, grandparent,* and so on appear to give more information than they do. They make me into a static noun. Even as starting points, they elide the questions that might allow you to see us as dynamic verbs: *What transition are you in the middle of? Where is your growing edge? What ambiguities do you live with? What has been emerging in your life over the past months? What do you do when you get up in the morning? How do you think about what it means to be healthy? What changes are you facing? What are you learning about yourself? What do you do with your grief? With humiliation?*

With frustration? How have your hopes shifted? How do you know the things you know? What do you make of inexplicable coincidences? I imagine being asked questions like these. I imagine what it would be like to focus in a clinical conversation with you, even briefly, on how I go about being the person I am being at this point in my life.

I can imagine even the kindest clinicians I know (you being one of them) rolling their eyes at the fanciful notion that there would ever be enough time to wander down such rabbit trails during a heavily scheduled day. But some do take a few steps down those paths. Some take those two minutes. It makes a difference.

I know neurologist and writer Oliver Sacks didn't have a typical practice, but he did much to open a place for imagination and human curiosity in the clinical encounter. His volumes of "clinical tales" record remarkable conversations with patients who presented with odd neurological disorders, fit no readily available categories, and engaged him in exhilarating medical detective work. He approached that work with a purposeful playfulness. Using one or more of a series of four questions, his basic approach to conversations with patients could be summarized in these queries: *Who are you? What is it like to be you? What are you already doing to deal with your condition? How can I help you?* Sacks seemed to understand his work as that of a trained witness who "came alongside" and assisted patients in devising strategies for functioning as fully and competently as they could. He approached them as people already traveling a learning curve, already having begun the healing work the body and mind do on their own. He treated them as people in the middle of a process that was often complex, subtle, and promising. He joined them in their efforts to cope, brought his considerable expertise to bear upon those efforts, and sometimes redirected them. But he always did so with a sense that something was already unfolding, emerging, verging. As I read about it, his practice sometimes seemed more like midwifery than any other form of medical intervention.

What would it mean for you to see me as a verb? Could it mean paying closer attention to your verbs and mine? Every verb opens a trailhead for further conversation: *I'm feeling, I'm noticing, I'm wondering, it's growing, it surfaces, it hurts, it recedes,* etc. You might choose any one of them for a little follow-up: *How does this feeling or shift come to your notice? In what situations do you find the pain growing worse? How does it hurt— does it ache? Burn? Throb? Pervade?* Pausing over a verb almost always leads to greater specificity, closer focus, and sharper attention to process. Some doctors use charts of up to fifty words for kinds and levels of pain to help expand patients' repertoire of options. This enables them to gather more nuanced, diagnostic information during the conversation. It's a vast improvement over the scale of one to ten.

As the list of possible verbs lengthens, a doctor and patient go beyond the staid, unmoving noun, and are much livelier and more willing to notice body, mind, and spirit in motion. Orderly and fixed as our innards may seem, we both know they're always fine-tuning, correcting, creating, eliminating, and healing. It's exhilarating to imagine all that's going on in this body quietly sitting here, masquerading as a noun. White blood cells are rushing to the site of a deep scratch on my arm. Stomach acids are working on the lovely salad I ate for lunch. Hormones are riding their version of messenger bikes through urban traffic carrying instructions about sleep, heart rate, and hunger. Cells are dividing and replacing their elders, diving into the work assigned, and living out their busy lives, generally with little fuss. Quietly they "endure their going hence, even as their coming hither." They ripen and die.

Every time I think about my own existence in these terms, I am amazed. I am busy *happening*. I am at least a participle—as much verb as noun—and able to be seen either way. Since we live in a culture that brands and commodifies everything in sight, turning even organic processes into possessions, it seems urgent that we help each other retrieve a sense of fluidity, of life happening before our very eyes, of spirit, light, and neutrinos dancing and moving about us and through us, and of divine energy whose name was once given as a verb: I am. I am being.

Buddhists recognize Buddha nature in all sentient beings, all of which are in a state of becoming. Hindu texts teach "Ether, air, fire, water, earth, planets, all creatures, directions, trees and plants, rivers and seas, they are all organs of God's body." Jews and Christians claim the Psalms that enjoin "everything that has life and breath" to praise the Creator. Trees clap their hands in those Psalms, and stormy winds move with intelligence and intention. In the Qur'an, as well as in the Bible, mountains, and fruit, trees, and small birds, and great sea creatures, and the oceans themselves participate in ongoing acts of emerging, coming forth, yielding, ripening, and returning to earth. However poetic and even fanciful these ways of speaking about life may become, it seems worth it to seriously consider that something is afoot. Something is going on—in us and around us—all the time, and our work is to get in step with it, hear its heartbeat, notice the forces at work and their direction, be open to the information that comes to us without ceasing, and learn to listen.

My Two Minutes: What keeps changing as you continue in medicine? How do you get unstuck?

Eating to Live

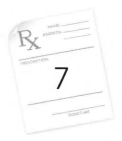

Real healthcare occurs outside of the doctor's office and hospitals, not when the patient shows up to make a complaint once their symptoms have developed.

—Emmanuel Fombu

Don't eat anything with more than five ingredients, or ingredients you can't pronounce.

—Michael Pollan

I will prevent disease whenever I can, for prevention is preferable to cure.

—2019 Version of the Hippocratic Oath

ONE OF THE THINGS that has made me proudest of my grandson is his decision to stop eating at McDonald's. He made it when he was fourteen years old after a conversation about how the company treats laborers, how beef production decimates rainforests, and what soft drinks do to teeth. He hasn't gone back. However, no doctor had told him these things.

Curiously, you don't ask much about what I eat unless my "presenting complaint" (a term I find irritating—see the chapter on language!) is directly related to my digestive tract. In fact, I'm astonished how few doctors have ever asked me what I eat. Or why I eat what I eat. Apart from vague reminders to "make healthy food choices," I haven't heard you mention pesticides, bovine growth hormone (BGH), genetically modified organisms (GMOs), the dangers of *E. coli* from factory farm runoff, or the side effects of food additives. I'm not sure why the Hippocratic teaching, "Let thy food be thy medicine," isn't recited at medical school graduations along with the Hippocratic oath to "do no harm." Anyway, I imagine this disturbing neglect of food matters isn't altogether your fault. Quite a few other people—patients and professionals—have mentioned the same strange omission. A 2015 article I read offers this bemusing research on the subject:

The Association of American Medical Colleges (AAMC) has recently declined to incorporate nutrition into their new blueprint for medical competencies. Furthermore, we have conducted three prior nutrition education surveys at four-year intervals since 2000 and consistently found that most medical schools do not even come close to the recommendation of the National Research Council to include at least 25–30 hours of nutrition education in the undergraduate medical curriculum.

I'm not laying blame at your doorstep; however, I am asking you to rise above your training and consider food as medicine. Continuing neglect of nutrition education is an "upstream" problem that affects those of us "downstream" who go to doctors like you for help with chronic diseases, ranging from daily fatigue to Type 2 diabetes, obesity, and a variety of inflammatory conditions that more consistent and informed attention to food could improve, if not heal.

Attention to nutrition seems more and more warranted in a food and drug system driven by profit and riddled with conflicts of interest. Finding affordable whole foods reasonably free of contaminants, sugar, preservatives, and other chemical additives has become a daunting project for me and many others with whom I've had this conversation. It makes weekly shopping a challenge, and I know that challenge is more difficult for people who live in food deserts on what Michael Pollan calls "food-like substances"—processed, preserved, packaged, and nearly devoid of nutritional value. I'm sure you see the "downstream" effects of the fake food epidemic every day. I'm also sure it wouldn't take more than a fraction of those extra two minutes to pass on Pollan's homely guidelines for good eating: "Eat real food. Not too much. Mostly vegetables." Or, even more briefly, "Don't eat anything that won't eventually rot."

I try not to do so. Thanks to books, articles, and documentaries by people I consider whistle-blowers on the massive corporations that profit from public ignorance and illness, I've cobbled together some helpful rules of thumb for grocery shopping and a repertoire of skeptical questions about prescription drugs and packaged cereals. I'd be happy to pass them on. It won't take me more than two minutes! Writers like John Robbins, Andrew Weil, Joshua Rosenthal, T. Colin Campbell, and Caldwell Esselstyn, and a growing collection of food documentaries from *Forks Over Knives* to *What the Health* to *Vegucated* to *Fed Up* have sharpened my awareness of how the food system works and how eating habits contribute to physical, mental, and spiritual health.

I'm grateful for this growing body of information becoming available, but it isn't routinely delivered, or even alluded to, in doctors' offices or hospitals, where nutritionists' advice seems so often to ignore the biggest elephant in the room by keeping the focus on individual choice and food groups rather than industrial processes. I'd love for people in the medical system to help me, my adult children, and my friends connect the dots between awareness of those processes, informed eating, and radiant well-being. Doing this kind of homework, I've learned about the surprising amount of protein in fresh peas, spinach, and kale; that glyphosate lingers in soil and on apple skins; and that there are half a dozen good reasons to avoid eating beef altogether. But I can't do the detailed blood work that might tell me what particular nutrients I'm missing and whether anything in my eating habits could explain occasional energy slumps.

I can go out of my insurance network to see a naturopath and pay out of pocket for nutritional guidance—and have done so. But I'd like you, my "primary care" physician, to help me with what seems "primary" among good health habits: eating consciously, carefully, and caringly, cultivating a relationship to food that will keep my body systems functioning properly and keep me in right relationship to the earth.

I'd like you to help me understand the key information on food labels, and clarify which of the additives listed in fine print might be harmful. I know aspartame is a neurotoxin, but I'd like you to unpack the implications of that sobering fact and maybe talk to me about the consequences of sugar (and sweetener) addiction. Because even knowing a few isolated scientific facts, it's hard to maintain a gold-standard awareness of what "healthy" means when so much that is unhealthy has been normalized by incessant, insidious marketing strategies: celebrity testimonies, eye-catching packaging, product placement, and the use of unprotected language like "healthy diet"—a term that can be bent to serve a variety of undeclared purposes.

I'd like you to help me understand what monosodium glutamate (MSG) does to brain pathways. I'd like you to help me understand why trans fats cause inflammation, or why food dyes are linked to chromosomal damage, or why my meat-eating friends need to avoid sodium nitrates. I think my curiosities on these matters are consequential. If I'm misinformed, I'd like to know that, too, and what counterevidence there may be. Whose claims are most credible, and why. I know you're not a chemistry teacher, but I believe one dimension of healing is teaching and one dimension of teaching is healing. Navigating the food system may be one of the most important—and neglected—issues in patient care. I'm a patient, and I care. So, if only by means of waiting-room brochures, or warnings, or recommended reading, I'd like your medical guidance to include the food factor.

And perhaps you need a little help from me. Maybe my questions will give you the incentive you need to seek out more continuing medical education about food, or cobble together a physicians' reading group on the subject. Maybe you wanted to take a nutrition course in med school and couldn't fit it into your schedule. Maybe you, too, feel constrained not only by time pressures that limit the scope of your reading, but also by the fact that much of the available research on food production, food additives, and food safety is funded by big players in the food industry. Maybe you've read the Center for Accountability in Science's recent report about the state of food and drug research:

Much of the research conducted into chemicals is performed by industry. Businesses have an interest in showing that their products are safe and employ more scientists than the government, non-profits, and universities combined. Industry also often collaborates with universities to conduct joint research or fund university-run research. And as with government, university, or non-profit-funded studies, industry-funded studies are often peer-reviewed and published in prestigious journals.

It's not uncommon for researchers to receive grants from private industry, non-profits, and governments throughout the course of their careers.

You and I inhabit the same incestuous food system. A decades-long trail of evidence suggests the Food and Drug Administration (FDA), big pharmaceutical companies, and major players in the food industry have consistently served each other's interests, often at the expense of risking public health. A *Time Magazine* report in 2016 spelled out the alarming extent to which the protection of industry profits has shaped government dietary guidelines for Americans. Dr. Robert Lustig from the University of California, San Francisco offered a summary statement in that report that gets at the heart of the problem: "Tasking the government agency that manages America's food production [the United States Department of Agriculture (USDA)] with crafting nutrition policy is akin to 'putting the fox in charge of the hen house.'"

So here we are in the hen house. How do we protect ourselves? We both eat. We both work in environments where there are doughnuts in the break room and Coke machines in the hallways. We both have families.

We're both target markets. We drive by the same neon-lit fast-food drive-throughs and see the same billboard ads for Absolut Vodka and Arby's. We frequent the same supermarkets—and perhaps, occasionally, peruse the shelves in health food stores. I'd like you to share my enthusiasm for food education, and perhaps a little salutary indignation over propaganda that makes it so hard to refuse juicy hamburgers, giant colas, or anything sweetened with high-fructose corn syrup.

To some extent, that means I'd like you to be willing to be political. Food is a political issue. If you go public with qualms about particular food products or processes, you could, of course, face real consequences. Nevertheless, some of your medical colleagues have done so. In 2016, a physicians committee at Grady Hospital in Atlanta, Georgia, sponsored three billboard ads challenging the hospital to go fast food free when its contract with McDonald's came up for renewal. This same group has publicized the problem of junk food in schools, the narcotic effects of cheese (which one doctor was quoted as calling it "dairy crack"), and the distressing reasons why Washington has not yet successfully curtailed the power of big food corporations to control research and publication, exert undue pressure on the FDA, and keep vital secrets from consumers.

It takes more than a village to confront the dubious practices in food production that endanger us all. The Physicians Committee for Responsible Medicine has about 150,000 members. The Center for Foodborne Illness Research and Prevention, the Consumer Federation of America, Consumers' Union, Food and Water Watch, the Partnership for Food Safety Education, and the Pew Charitable Trust Health Network are among numerous organizations that work together and independently in their various niches to ensure food safety and food security. I'm grateful for every one of those who have directed their efforts toward those ends. I'd like to swell their ranks. I'd like for you to, as well.

I also need your help owning up to my unhealthier eating habits and changing them where necessary. It matters to me that you be morally, as well as politically, engaged in this effort. I want you to be committed, as I am becoming committed, to the idea that how I care for my body, and how you do, are not morally neutral matters. In fact, I believe moral neutrality is no more acceptable on matters of food consumption than it is on matters of sex and reproductive rights, or allocation of public health care funding (such as it is). There may be painful ambiguities involved and forces beyond any of our control, but we have a right to know how our food is produced, at whose cost, with what effects on the ecosystems, compromised by what contaminants, how much petroleum it used to get to me, and how it affects my arterial walls, or microbiome or hormonal balance. You can help inform me on these matters while you also inform yourself. I wish you, as I wish my family and myself, in the most literal sense, *bon appétit.*

My Two Minutes: What are your own food practices? What basic decisions have you made about food?

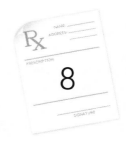

HIGHER POWER

Prayer . . . offers many of the same health and stress-relief benefits as meditation. Some of these benefits include reduced feelings of stress, lower cholesterol levels, improved sleep, reduced anxiety and depression, fewer headaches, more relaxed muscles, and longer life spans.

—DANIEL G. AMEN

Not to employ prayer with my patients was the equivalent of deliberately withholding a potent drug or surgical procedure.

—LARRY DOSSEY

Above all, I must not play at God.
—2019 VERSION OF THE HIPPOCRATIC OATH

LAST TIME I MENTIONED praying for a friend's recovery, we lost eye contact. You began peering at the computer screen and changed the subject. As I have come to understand, you're no more comfortable broaching the matter of spirituality—certainly not of prayer—than most doctors. I don't blame you. "Prayer" is a word that's been contaminated by association with oversimplified, magical thinking and hyperbolic televangelistic fervor. My favorite way of thinking of prayer is simply "the practice of the presence of God"—a phrase that bears wide, generous interpretation and application. To speak of prayer is perhaps, after all, just a way of saying I'm open to mystery. I watch for it. I welcome it. I hope you do too.

But except for those who attended religiously affiliated medical schools, most of you folks have had little encouragement to reflect on spirituality in your education or training. The oversimplified notion that spirituality and science are somehow at odds, or even mutually exclusive, continues to affect both patients' expectations and doctors' behaviors—even though top-level scientists from major faith traditions (Albert Einstein, Francis Collins, Bruno Guiderdoni, and Freeman Dyson among them) see them as convergent. As one doctor put it, "It took a lot of time to establish medicine as a legitimate science, and we don't want to lose that credibility." I get it, but that concern seems unnecessarily defensive. I'm not sure how people who don't pray imagine prayer, but they might be surprised at the range of experience that word covers.

I've taken enough science courses to understand the value of the empirical method and double-blind experiments and the reasons for focusing on measurable, repeatable results. Nevertheless, seeing a growing number of reports on the effects of meditation, spirituality, and faith as factors in health, even in scientific journals, gratifies me. Conversation about those factors seems to be more permissible, at least in some professional circles, than it was a few decades ago. Nevertheless, some of the best doctors I know, you included, continue to roll your eyes surreptitiously or redirect when the subject arises. Or make small concessions that "some people" may find their faith helpful and leave it at that. One article posted on WebMD, however, claims that research focusing on the power of prayer in healing has nearly doubled over the past twenty years.

Some things, by definition, cannot be scientifically studied. As Horatio reminds Hamlet, there are "more things in heaven and earth . . . than are dreamt of in your philosophy," and certainly more, I would add, than can be counted, measured, or submitted to academic journals.

Don't you get curious, though, about what lies just outside the boundaries of a strictly controlled experiment? Or wonder what to make of a one-off occurrence—say an inexplicable, against-the-odds recovery—you can't explain? Or what to do with an account of visions or prescient dreams by a perfectly credible person? And don't you wonder what actually happens when people meditate or pray?

I wonder what room could be made in professional medical conversation to reflect on the inexplicable, mysterious singular event. I wonder what you do with a patient who claims an angel appeared and helped. I wonder what place anecdotal evidence could have in "evidence-based" medicine. Even though people's stories about their spiritual or mystical or paranormal experiences can be riddled with ulterior motives, there are enough of them for me to think some portion of those testimonies deserves serious consideration. Listening closely to those stories might enable both you and your patients to explore how subtle guidance or renewed energy or hope changes the course of recovery. They seem like usable information.

These days, I think often about how spiritual practice may be one of the keys to healing, wholeness, and good health, remembering as I do that "whole" and "holy" share a taproot. If—or when—I find myself in a hospital, I'd like to know that my doctor—not just the chaplain—could acknowledge my spiritual needs and the spiritual dimension of my illness and healing as part of the story. I remember one conversation in which a medical student, presented with the possibility that he might have to serve as a chaplain stand-in for a dying patient, immediately and emphatically insisted, "That's not my job." As the conversation progressed, though, he reflected that at some point, in some critical moment, it could be. I would hope that, if you're mentoring younger colleagues, you'd broach the ways spirituality and health might be intertwined.

As a hospice volunteer, which no doubt is easier than as a doctor whose professional circles might be heavily populated by skeptics, I can pay attention to dimensions of patient experience that are both physical and spiritual. Both are more sharply outlined near the end of life. I pray for patients; occasionally, if they wish, I pray with them. I believe prayer actually draws and directs divine energy in mysterious, powerful ways. Having grown up in a devout family for whom daily prayer, Wednesday-night prayer meetings, and church on Sundays were a deeply entrenched part of life, I've heard so many stories about answers to prayer that I can't dismiss prayer as an instrument of healing even though my particular faith understanding has branched rather far from that of my childhood church. In fact, as my faith journey has taken me into unexpected places, some of them dark and dry, some luminous and surprising, prayer has become both more mysterious and more ordinary—sometimes not very different from pausing to breathe deeply before returning to the present moment.

Popular Franciscan writer Richard Rohr says, "Holiness is simply being connected to our Source." Whether we understand that Source as a God whose "center is everywhere" or the life force encoded in DNA, it seems reasonable to recognize a realm of mystery that lies just beyond what the most powerful electron microscopes can reveal. And it's always seemed to me, dear doctor, that you're a reasonable person.

One of the best stories I've heard about prayer and illness in recent years came from a friend who is a pastor. As he engaged his congregation in exploring what gifts each of them brought to the community and how the community might receive and foster them, one very quiet woman approached him and asked if she could accompany him on his visits to the hospital. When he took her, she asked if she could pray with the patients. After some weeks of this, he noticed that people improved once she prayed. Some became more peaceful, some more hopeful, and some actually physically better. Finally, he asked her what was happening. She replied that she'd always sensed she had a gift of healing, but didn't know what to do with it or how to share it.

None of us knows exactly how prayer "works" any more than we know how subatomic particles respond to each other at great distances, but its effects seem clear to me. Those who dismiss its value have to overlook a mountain of evidence and many truly surprising stories. I don't think you're among those who are dismissive, but you do sidestep the conversation when you can.

Be assured I'm not asking you to pray with me. That's likely a bridge too far. Maybe venturing into that territory makes you feel like the one in the thin gown in a cold room waiting uneasily for a conversation you're not sure you want to have. Still, there's reason to have it. I'm in pretty good company in believing that prayer, as well as meditation, chant, and other healing spiritual practices, should be seriously considered in healing and health. A simple internet search brings up multiple academic articles citing the positive effects of prayer or meditation on healing and recovery in controlled studies, though many of them also acknowledge the limitations inherent in trying to study mystical experience empirically. One of them opens simply with this claim: "Evidence . . . suggests that certain spiritual beliefs and the practice of prayer are associated with improved coping and better health outcomes." Another concludes:

> Most studies have shown that religious involvement and spirituality are associated with better health outcomes, including greater longevity, coping skills and health-related quality of life (even during terminal illness) and less anxiety, depression and suicide. Several studies have shown that addressing the spiritual needs of the patient may enhance recovery from illness.

There are plenty of skeptical responses to these claims, but I find the growing body of studies like these both intriguing and encouraging. Take a look. Let me know what you think. A two-minute exchange on the subject could be life-giving for both of us.

Healing traditions in so many cultures include these kinds of practices, it seems parochial not at least to be curious about what shamans have done and still do, or about the many stories of the mysterious, sudden appearances of people who help and heal and then disappear. Dipping into these kinds of accounts one can at least speculate about some of the ways body, mind, and spirit are knit together. Begin, perhaps, with studies of psychosomatic illness and then stretch from there into accounts of healings attributed directly to some kind of spiritual intervention like the laying on of hands. You don't have to go back to ancient texts to find them; testimonies to enigmatic kinds of healing are so abundant it takes a fortress-like bureaucracy to keep them from seeping into research labs, and classrooms, and clinics.

But maybe, after all this, I've misconstrued your hesitations. Maybe you *do* pray, meditate, practice Reiki or sacred dance, or read about shamanism. If so and we've never talked about that, I would love to know, at least a little, what you think about those matters, and how they help shape your understanding of patient care. As a physician, you are in a privileged position to witness not only the well-documented physiological processes we call healing, but also, no doubt, kinds of transformation that don't lend themselves so easily to empirical testing. If you're willing to share a bit, I'd love to know what mysteries you've seen and contemplated.

I know doctors who pray with patients, some at the risk of professional censure. I suppose it's easier to do if one works in a faith-based hospital setting, or mission clinic, or in palliative care. But if you don't pray aloud with patients, do you think having some quiet practice—e.g., posting a prayer or the words to the Metta meditation on the wall, or, if music is part of the work environment, a quiet, slow chant—might not enhance and enrich your healing work? I know it would deepen the relaxation, and openness and peace with which I could participate in my own healing.

Resistances run deep. Many people have been hurt by religion or by pushy, pious people, and don't want to mix spirituality and medicine any more than they want to hear politics from the pulpit. But that mingling seems inevitable to me, as it also seems inevitable that illness or serious injury will stir spiritual longings or unsettling questions about what might be, as the Heidelberg catechism puts it, "our only comfort in life and death."

Your resistances, whatever they are, may have been reinforced by the insistence on an empirical, scientific, double-blind, thoroughly vetted, strictly professional approach to inquiry you probably received in medical school. It has seemed to me, just as an observer, that precisely because medicine isn't an exact science, because good medicine requires compassion and intuition and even improvisation at times, some doctors cling all the harder to scientific standards and eschew the rest. But not the good ones, among whom I'd hope you count yourself. I imagine if I asked you to tell stories about the mysteries you've encountered in medicine, if you let memories gather around that word, you'd have more than a few stories to tell.

When I say I pray, it doesn't necessarily mean bowing my head and addressing God by a particular name, though I like experimenting with the names of God—how each one invites the imagination in a different way: Father-Mother-God, Spirit, Source, Creator, Holy One, Comforter, "Heart of my own heart." And when I say I pray, it means that the habit of prayer has gradually become like the habits of breathing or eating. The day doesn't happen without it. So it must be taken into account.

In a spirit of prayerfulness, then, which is not far from playfulness, let me suggest how you might best help me and other patients who pray. You might ask about what shores up the inner resources I bring to healing. You might collect and pass along simple meditation practices other patients have found helpful. You might post a simple prayer or an affirmation or "May the Force be with you" somewhere visible in your office so that while we wait, chilly in our white paper gowns, we might gaze at something more inspiring than a map of the nervous system. Or you might, as I leave, assure me in your own words that you will, as the Quakers say, "hold me in the light."

My Two Minutes: How do you seek guidance? What does your own spirituality have to do with your work in medicine? What helps you when it gets discouraging?

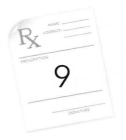

FEAR HAPPENS

Be afraid. Be very afraid.

—DICKENS

Be not afraid.

—JESUS

DESPITE MY EFFORTS IN the previous chapters to sound like your peer and to remind you that I'm a professional with a certain academic distance on my own and others' conditions, let me acknowledge here a darker truth: illness is scary. Serious illness is terrifying. No matter how much I've educated myself, the prospect of developing a serious illness—especially if it diminishes mental functions—remains mysterious and threatening. Sometimes, no matter how nice you are, just walking through your office door is scary: who knows what dire news you might deliver after perusing the most recent printout of my blood work or the routine X-ray I took to renew my contract at work?

Suppressing my own apprehensions, I've watched friends, family members, students, colleagues, and people on the street coping with conditions I can't imagine handling with the grace or courage I see in them: multiple sclerosis that laces the smallest physical tasks with frustration; the slowing, debilitating shake of Parkinson's; chronic back pain that is only partially relieved by icing, pillows, drugs, immersion in pools, and meditation; cancer with all the attendant dismaying losses of hair, energy, work, appetite, sound sleep, and a sense of the future altered, even for those with every hope of "cure." How do they face the morning? How would I?

One friend of mine—a gifted storyteller with a wry sense of humor and an astute political mind, an activist and energetic teacher for decades—now spends her days in a wheelchair and her nights in a recliner. She uses a walker to get to the bathroom—a little trip she has to plan and time carefully, since falling would be a major problem. She uses a metal "grabber" to pick things up off the floor since she can't bend far. Her joints ache. She sleeps fitfully. And while she remains one of the most engaging conversationalists I know, she has to do most of her visiting at home because leaving her carefully equipped living space, even to go to the doctor's office, uses up a day's worth of energy. I don't know how she sustains her good spirits. They're not fake, but I suspect they are punctuated by some very dark nights. I wonder what she does with her fear. She doesn't go there. I don't ask.

Another friend is waking every day to the slow encroachment of dementia. He pauses in doorways, uncertain about where he's going. He gets lost on familiar walks. He repeats stories he can't remember having told an hour ago. He is learning to mask his confusions, and doing well at it because he's smart, but I'm guessing the mask covers some very scary moments.

Another friend died recently, but not before she lost most of her sight and nearly all of her hearing, mobility, and appetite. We communicated by means of a small whiteboard on which I wrote in large letters. It was arduous and limiting. Her patience with the process exceeded mine, though just being in her company taught me much about humility and grace. And her wit made me think humor should have a high place on any list of spiritual gifts. It was certainly a gift to me.

I've watched these people with amazement as well as an aching heart. I've also watched those who love them, who witness such losses at close range—faithful caregivers who reorganized their daily routines around others' pressing (and sometimes unappealing) needs, whose own anguish and anger are veiled for the sake of kindness, and who have had to find their own ways to cope with emotional exhaustion. Watching them, I wonder how they manage their own anxieties. I wonder how you manage yours. You see so many of the "ills that flesh is heir to." You have learned to maintain a "clinical distance" on most of them, though I imagine there are nights when you go home filled with sorrow or dread. "We strive to put away from us / That which terrorizes the heart," Norman Macleod writes, but even as I remember that line, another comes to mind, written by Annie Stenzel, a poet newly diagnosed with multiple sclerosis: "Terror / is all I am."

Some fears are, of course, a normal response to the world we live in. More and more young people, aware of geopolitical tensions and climate change, struggle with deep depression and chronic anxiety, not to mention those who live in war zones or conditions of relentless poverty where danger is real and present and daily. A recent report from Harvard Medical School clearly acknowledges what I imagine we all intuitively know: the anxieties many suffer (if they haven't had their heads in the sand) lie at the root of a whole range of physical and mental illnesses. The folks at Harvard offer some hope in both "cognitive-behavioral therapies" and anti-anxiety drugs. Whether we pathologize it or spiritualize it, whether we dose it or let it drive us to our knees—or to eating, drinking, and making merry in "desperate gaiety"—fear remains a challenge.

I know, and want you to know, that some days fear finds its way through even my strongest defenses. I am afraid of what my next years will bring, not to mention the coming decade of new and unsettling "normals." I am not particularly afraid of death, but I am of the range of afflictions that could precede it: dwindling energy, repeated bereavements, pain, bewilderment, powerlessness. No matter how firmly I cling to a faith that sustains me, I find that my breath goes shallow and my heart starts to race, and I scroll through my address book while asking myself what kindly friend might welcome a call for comfort in the middle of working—or sleeping—hours. I don't want to suggest that my fears are diagnosable pathologies; I have coping strategies and access to love that generally casts out fear before its roots drive too deep. But fear comes unbidden, often in the night, and assails me.

Psalms comfort me, as does my husband's voice, and sometimes a voice or two from Comedy Central. When fear tightens its grip, a centering word or phrase can open interior prayer space: "Abba" or "Peace" or "Be with me." Poetry helps—Donne's "Hymn to God in My Sickness," for instance, which, after detailing his besetting fears, ends, "I fear no more," or Hopkins's image of the Holy Ghost brooding "over the bent world"— smeared and grayed by industrial pollutants—with "bright wings." Or Wendell Berry's lovely poem, "The Peace of Wild Things," which moves from confession of fear to a kind of absolution of it in "the grace of the world." Its opening lines take me to a very familiar place and state of mind:

> When despair for the world grows in me
> and I wake in the night at the least sound
> in fear of what my life and my children's lives
>   may be,
> I go and lie down where the wood drake
> rests in his beauty on the water, and the great
>   heron feeds.
> I come into the peace of wild things
> who do not tax their lives with forethought
> of grief . . .

Unlike Berry, I don't live in rural Kentucky, though I do live near a river where consoling walks can be taken and a little birdsong, as well as an occasional chorus of frogs, can be heard. Like him, I do wake with fears that drive me to those places where I can be among creatures who, as he so beautifully puts it, "do not tax their lives with forethought of grief." I find consolation in considering the lilies when I can get to the lilies. Maybe I should plant a few lilies, just to consider them. The need for consolation comes again and again. Sorrows arise and linger and don't quite leave. Sometimes they merely flicker. Sometimes they stay for a whole season while those lilies hibernate in their bulbs under the frost.

You, who spend so much time in what Susan Sontag called "the kingdom of the sick," see more fear and anxiety in a day than most. I wonder if someone in med school taught you what students at Brown University School of Medicine are being taught now: to include a "spiritual assessment" in patient interviews that begins with the question, "I'm wondering, where do you find comfort or hope in this time of illness? When things get tough, what keeps you going?"

It may be a good thing for both of us that you're not the one I rely on for spiritual comfort, but one day you might be if the chaplain's not there, and my family has gone home, and night is looming after your last rounds. I hope

I can count on you for a comforting word, full eye contact, and a healing touch. I hope you're not afraid of my fear.

I've seen doctors who are. I remember one who stood across the large room, hovering in the doorway as if ready to escape, while a young woman I loved begged him to say something clear that might help her make the excruciating decision to take her dying husband off the ventilator that was likely at that point a futile measure. He made no eye contact. He gazed at the monitors and recited what he saw there—information that hadn't varied much for days. He didn't address her by name. He was, I imagine, struggling with his own fear of legal repercussions if he said anything that sounded like a directive to terminate a life. But what I saw was his fear amplifying hers. It was tragic. She finally made the decision. I sat with her while she held her husband who quietly and quickly died. The death itself was not fearsome—just deeply sad.

One often hears that love is the opposite of fear, perhaps so often it seems cliché. But like most clichés, it has become one because it's true. Loving words allay fear. Loving presence can dispel it. Love—not particular affection, but the force we channel when we're open to the Source that gives us our common life and breath—is what heals "all our diseases," as we live and as we die. Fear is one of those.

My Two Minutes: What's scariest about your work with patients? How do you handle your own fears?

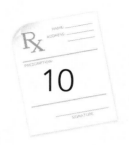

Ripeness Is All

Men must endure
Their going hence, even as their coming hither:
Ripeness is all.

—King Lear, Act V, Scene 2

I will apply, for the benefit of the sick, all measures
[that] are required, avoiding those twin traps of
overtreatment and therapeutic nihilism.

—2019 Version of the Hippocratic Oath

I'VE OFTEN SAID TO the younger people in my life—
students, kids, grandkids—"You never know what you're
being prepared for." I don't, either. But these days, I
find myself more conscious of making myself ready
for what comes with aging and dying, especially, after

recently having the conversation with you as I filled out my "Advance Health Care Directives" form, and then again with my "Five Last Wishes" form. I'm glad these forms and conversations have entered into routine care. I've seen what happens in some families when final wishes aren't made clear. I want to be ready when the time comes. But at a deeper level, the kind of readiness I hope for is a sustained, clear willingness to walk the final stretch of my path consciously and thoughtfully, prepared to accept responsibility for decisions along the way about medications, remediations, and relinquishments, and new habits.

With increasing pertinence as age comes upon me, I see how readiness to die is a measure of the capacity to live each day with gratitude, presence, and joy. I've learned what that can look like from hospice patients who face their situations with sidelong humor or resignation or the consolations of small things—flowers or a good dinner. I've also learned about it from a dear friend and former professor who spent a good part of her early youth in concentration camps. After the war she wrote a poem, "A Colloquy with the Angel of Death," where she addresses Death with wry acceptance as "Old friend, old adversary." She said to me once that when you had come face to face with death and walked away, you were free, indeed.

That kind of freedom is its own kind of healing. I wonder if you've ever thought about your work as setting patients free. I'm sure you've witnessed remarkable changes in those who have become free of the fear of death. I know those changes come from "near-death experiences" sometimes. I've found many of those accounts both fascinating and consoling. I hope you read some. I'd love to use one of our two minutes debriefing one of those stories. Almost all who return from afterlife excursions have a deepened sense of purpose in being here and no fear of death. You may be a skeptic; you may believe these accounts lie too far outside the parameters of evidence you are trained (or allowed) to validate as credible. I find such stories helpful, though, and I'd love to see you open a small window, if not a door, to reflect on what happens in that mysterious space where life borders death. I'll give you a few of my favorite titles, if you ask. Maybe even if you don't.

I've looked to the mystics and philosophers and poets from various generations and traditions to help me see how readiness to die can, paradoxically, help us "choose life" and enter into it with more exuberance, playfulness, and abandon.

I don't like euphemistic language that glosses over the realities of loss, pain, and even terror with superficial pieties, or encourages false cheerfulness about aging and death. But I do like "ripening." It reminds me of the cycle of life and death in which we find ourselves, which is neither good nor bad, but, as *King Lear* suggests, a maturity that fully accepts mortality, uncertainty, and the conditions on which life is given and taken, as well as the risks it entails. I want to age with this kind of maturity and acceptance. I want to go when the time comes. I don't want to outlive myself.

I know you're trained to "save" lives. I know in many cases, this becomes a matter of prolonging life despite the pain, loss of function, or even loss of any evident capacity for enjoyment or awareness. All of us in the US grew up in a health care system that has prided itself on aggressive interventions that can effectively cure or "manage" diseases. But its emphasis on intervention has de-emphasized both prevention of disease before it happens and preparation for death. The latter, in particular, is hard to foster in a system that constructs death as a failure to cure—a negative outcome, a consummation devoutly to be avoided. It's often those who work in palliative care or in hospice organizations, caring for those with terminal illnesses in their final days, who most clearly understand that the line that divides care of the body and care of the soul can blur. Hospice organizations seem more oriented toward integrating those two dimensions of care than most hospitals.

As long as death is the ultimate enemy of those who practice medicine, I don't imagine I'll get much help from conventional care in preparing and hoping for a gracious and timely death. But perhaps, despite the short shrift your med school may have given to helping you help us die well, you find yourself interested in doing that. Assuming you are, in fact, interested, let me offer you a very short list of my own hopes for a good and humane death. I hope you will help me pursue these aims as I prepare for the next season of life.

1. I hope to go when it's time. Knowing when "my time has come" isn't as easy as it once was since there are so many ways now to prolong life and postpone death. I don't think "postponing death" is the same as "prolonging life." In her powerful poem, "Death Psalm: O Lord of Mysteries," Denise Levertov lists the ways an aged woman has "made ready to die":

> She grew old.
> She made ready to die.
> She gave counsel to women and men, to young
>   girls and young boys.
> She remembered her griefs.
> She remembered her happinesses.

She watered the garden.
She accused herself.
She forgave herself.
She learned new fragments of wisdom.
She forgot old fragments of wisdom.
She abandoned certain angers.
She gave away gold and precious stones.
She counted-over her handkerchiefs of fine lawn.
She continued to laugh on some days, to cry on
    others,
unfolding the design of her identity.
She practiced the songs she knew, her voice
gone out of tune
but the breathing-pattern perfected.
She told her sons and daughters she was ready.
She maintained her readiness.
She grew very old.
She watched the generations increase.
She watched the passing of seasons and years.

This is the first half of the poem. The second half begins with the line, "She did not die." It continues with painful images of a woman lying "half-speechless, incontinent, / aching in body, wandering in mind" with a "plastic tube taped to her nose" and concludes with an outcry to the "Lord of mysteries" on behalf of those whose readiness to die, whose "ancient, / courteously waiting life" seems to have been overlooked by whoever comes to take weary pilgrims home. Her "waiting" reflects what seems to me a very common contemporary bafflement over how to handle end-of-life decisions now that death can be so effectually, if not wisely or graciously, postponed. Grace matters to me, which brings me to the second item on my list:

2. I hope to go with grace. Stirring as it is, I don't find much personal inspiration in Dylan Thomas's "Do Not Go Gentle into That Good Night." "Gentle" sounds good to me. I don't want to "rage against the dying of the light," but to watch it come the way I have recently taken to watching sunsets, their changing colors, the way evening light suffuses full summer trees, the way shades of flame gather at the horizon and comes the way Emily Dickinson saw dawn break: "a ribbon at a time." I read Jane Kenyon's poem "Let Evening Come," as a kind of prayer for the grace I hope for in others' deaths and in my own: not simply an acquiescence, but rather a slow, attentive greeting of each harbinger of transition: light moving on bales of hay, crickets "chafing," dew collecting on grass, the fox returning to "its sandy den," the shed going black. Rather than a litany of loss, she offers a slow, lyrical acknowledgment of the beauties specific to day's end, concluding with resonant lines I take as both instruction and a word of deep consolation as I think about my own death and the deaths of those I love, as well as those I see as hospice patients, with each one of whom I have learned something about how many ways there are of "going forth": "Let it come, as it will, and don't / be afraid. God does not leave us / comfortless, so let evening come." There is power in that word, "let," as well as permission, and consent, and intention. It is a way of claiming and owning what must and will be. Kenyon's poem has been a gift to me, so I share it with you here. I may even share it again when my time comes, reminding you that the dying have gifts to give. I have received them again and again as I have witnessed others' going. So, I add this third item to my list of hopes:

3. I hope to die in a way that may be a gift to those who love me. My mother's death was like that. She lived longer than she may have hoped, having often said she wanted to go when she was "no longer useful." But we had some sweet conversations about not being useful in those final months, in which I was given a chance to express, as I hadn't before, how much gratitude I felt for her "human merely being," as e. e. cummings put it.

When I think how my children may have to watch me go, and may have to care for me in ways I'd rather not have to be cared for, it's good for me to remember the gift of my mother's ninety-fourth year—her patient going, how her laughter survived cognitive losses, how firmly she held my hand as we talked. And I imagine they, and I, may have chances to consent to whatever comes, ready or not, and in those opportunities find occasions for growth that are, in themselves, gifts.

Your work may be done by that time. You may have handed me over to the care of a hospice doctor, or my family. I may simply have refused further interventions. But if you're around and watching, I hope you'll recognize "ripeness" when it arrives, and allow the fruit to fall, or be plucked, in due time.

My Two Minutes: What's the most important thing you've learned about end-of-life care? About how to talk about dying? What have the dying taught you?

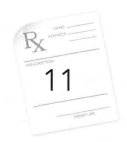

ENTERTAINING ALTERNATIVES

> Medication, surgery, and radiation are the weapons with which conventional medicine foolishly shoots the messengers called symptoms.
>
> —MOKOKOMA MOKHONOANA

> I will not be ashamed to say "I know not," nor will I fail to call in my colleagues when the skills of another are needed for a patient's recovery.
>
> —2019 VERSION OF THE HIPPOCRATIC OATH

I have to laugh when people ask me if I do alternative, herbal, or holistic medicine. "No," I reply. "We do state-of-the-art medicine. In other words, we find the biochemical, nutritional and environmental causes and cures rather than blindly drugging everything. Sure, herbs are gentler, safer and more physiologic than drugs and holistic medicine attempts to incorporate many diverse modalities, etc. But there is no substitute for finding the underlying biochemical causes and cures. This is real medicine. This is where medicine should and would have been decades ago, if it had not been abducted by the pharmaceutical industry."

—SHERRY A. ROGERS, *DETOXIFY OR DIE*

When you drink ayahuasca, and you get to see divinity, you can almost never speak of it because it's too big for words.

—GERARD ARMOND POWELL

THANK YOU FOR YOUR referral to the acupuncturist. I'll let you know how it went after I've completed the twelve sessions my insurance plan covers. Even though you occasionally find amusement in my "food fads" (I see you smiling to yourself when I remind you I don't eat meat and avoid gluten), and even though you may be slightly annoyed when I acknowledge that I also see a naturopath, I think you also see that antibiotics and acupuncture have both helped me. I am a grateful recipient of childhood vaccinations and also a contented and generally healthy vegetarian. I'm interested in what doctors can teach me about insulin response, serotonin reuptake inhibitors, and beta blockers. I'm also interested in reports and studies about the benefits of meditation, prayer, deep relaxation, as well as in what we can learn from people who have experimented with holotropic breathing or visited Ayurvedic practitioners or undergone a "near-death experience."

I am also aware that medicine as taught and practiced in most American hospitals and medical schools is heavily influenced and even constrained by research funding from giant pharmaceutical companies and food industries. I'd like to understand how other approaches work because there's much evidence that, to varying degrees, they do work. I don't dismiss "Western medicine"; I'm just curious about what benefits may lie in alternatives. When I seek healing elsewhere, it's not out of personal dissatisfaction with your care. It's because there's more help to be had that I can't access in your office, no matter how sympathetic you may be to my curiosities.

I've mentioned this to you before, but I am more than a little concerned that medicine is politicized on a historically unprecedented scale: the FDA, USDA, AMA, and big pharmaceutical companies with their very big lobbying budgets have done a lot of cross-pollinating. I'm aware that healing methods with deep roots in other cultures, that emerge from spiritual practices and traditions, that are not easily verifiable by standard double-blind empirical testing, and that don't promise profit tend to be underreported, marginalized, and sometimes suppressed in the public press and in professional journals. I also know, as one writer put it, "Many of those in the medical fraternity instantly label treatments in the traditional, natural or holistic health fields as quackery. This word is even used to describe Traditional Chinese Medicine and the Indian Ayurveda, two medical systems which are far older than Western-European medicine and globally just as popular."

As you know, medicine has always had an interdependent but uneasy relationship with faith traditions and psychic, energetic, or spiritual healers. Even "evidence-based" medicine as recognized by the AMA and state licensing boards is beholden to its own dogma about what is acceptable "evidence." That's a double-bind, if you ask me. I've met doctors who are openly interested in energetic healing, therapeutic touch, Chinese herbal or Indian Ayurvedic medicine, or even chiropractic or naturopathy who pay a professional cost for venturing into those borderlands where strictly scientific ways of knowing are challenged by medical intuitionists, shamans, yogis, and many quiet individuals who find they have a gift of healing through prayer or presence that can't be fully understood.

The best scientists I know (and it's been my privilege to count many practicing scientists and good doctors like you as my friends) do their work with a quality of attention and enthusiasm that seems infused with Spirit. Certainly, the role of dreams, intuitive leaps, epiphanies, and sidelong, "right-brained" routes to insight have their place—and not a small one—in the history of science. I think of Archimedes leaping out of his bathtub, having suddenly connected new dots and understood how to measure volume. Or Newton and the apple. Or Einstein's dream. According to one survey, "Seventy-two of eighty-three Nobel Laureates in science and medicine all implicated intuition in their success."

There are, to reference Hamlet again, more things in heaven and on earth than are allowed for in standard American medicine or in the pages of AMA-approved medical journals. I want you to know I have benefited from some of these "more things." My migraines, and later a peptic ulcer, improved significantly after biofeedback training, which I took when drugs failed.

Acupuncture sessions have taken me into what I would describe as an altered state, so deep was the experience of relaxation and inner quiet they enabled. A month-long "detox" regimen prescribed by a naturopath restored my flagging energies dramatically. And every morning, even a short period of meditation seems to enhance the cognitive clarity I carry into the day. And yet, I hasten to add, I am aware alternative approaches to health and healing have their own pitfalls; anything subtle can be oversimplified. Eula Biss makes this point about the notion of "natural": "The use of 'natural' as a synonym for 'good' is almost certainly a product of our profound alienation from the natural world." In other words, I get the counterpoint you seem to want to make, that natural alternatives to synthetic drugs aren't a simple or quick fix to the excesses of for-profit pharmaceuticals' domination of medicine.

Having talked at length with practitioners of integrative or complementary medicine, I know something about their frustration with the ways their work can be romanticized and expropriated by marketers willing to prey on a gullible public. I respect their courage in taking a medical path less traveled in this culture and the remarkable underreported successes that sustain their decisions to remain on that path. I just wish your paths crossed more often.

And notice: here I am on your appointment calendar because I also want you to know I recognize the irreplaceable value of what you do. I need you to look down my throat and into my ear and probe my belly and notice small lesions that might be significant. I need you to send me to the otolaryngologist, or the neurologist, or the gastroenterologist and remind me when it's time for the dreaded colonoscopy or mammogram (not that I won't drag my feet or need to be reminded more than once when that time comes). I'd like you and my other practitioners to know about each other. I'd like to see you at that learning edge in the medical conversation that is becoming more hospitable and inclusive, more widely "integrative," and more open to new kinds of evidence and discussion of unusual healing experiences than it has been for most of my life.

I mentioned that I see a naturopath who has helped me fine-tune and balance my eating habits and navigate our confusing, corporately dominated food system in ways that protect and enhance my general health and well-being. I don't remember when an MD has asked me what I eat unless the presenting complaint was an ulcer or a specific digestive problem. I don't remember a doctor's ever suggesting that I be aware of (and wary of) chemical additives, or pesticides, or high-fructose corn syrup. My naturopath takes clients on field trips through the local supermarket to help us develop usable, specific criteria for genuinely healthy food choices by learning how to read labels and recognize how many health claims are unregulated marketing messages. We learn how much "health food" isn't. From that same naturopath, I've benefited from conversations about how inflammation lies at the root of many diseases and what an anti-inflammatory diet looks like—a lot like the simple diet of whole foods my grandparents ate. (I like Michael Pollan's general advice not to eat food products with ingredients your grandmother wouldn't recognize.)

I also find it helpful to talk with the chiropractor I see occasionally about the importance of body align- ment and its relationship to preventing inflammation and compression. My chiropractor's attention not only to the position of my vertebrae, but also to the psychosomatic factors affecting posture, to proper adjustment of the lenses in my glasses, and to the ergonomics of my work- place (still working on this one; I like to write in an easy chair with my laptop on my lap) has been of real practical help. Conversations with her have a different focus and set of assumptions from conversations with any MD I've seen—complementary, usually, rather than conflicting.

I like the term "complementary medicine" better than "alternative medicine." I like medical ecumenism.

I was delighted when a doctor I saw recommended not only a medication for a specific condition, but also mineral supplements and—as she wrote boldly on a prescription pad—"two days in bed with a good book." There is no substitute for rest, she insisted. The body wants to heal itself. You have to give it a chance to do that.

The best experience I ever had with a skilled acupuncturist took me to a place of profound relaxation, out of the pain I walked in with, and into what I can only describe as an altered state of consciousness. During our sessions, I came to recognize how blocked energy can flow again, and how "flow" feels—open, awake, alive.

I read around about Eastern medical practices and became respectfully aware of how deeply medical traditions are rooted in cultural assumptions. I began to examine my own assumptions and to reckon with my own felt experience in new terms. I wonder if you do that now and then. I'd love to hear your two minutes on medicine and culture!

I began reading about chakras, and energetic healing, and psychic healing. I began to experience the benefits of meditation and even the elementary-level practices of qi gong and yoga I explored.

It doesn't take a long search on the internet to see how many questionable sites offer approaches to healing that look a lot like an amateur healer's self-promotion. But there are also many serious-minded, scholarly, thoughtful, credentialed, and experienced people who have risked a great deal professionally and personally to pursue avenues of healing that emerge from wisdom traditions that lie outside the parameters of conventional Western medicine. Some of those healing modalities entail faith practices. Some of them use the arts as instruments of awareness. Most embrace the reality of the numinous, since the mind-body-spirit relationship can't be measured and assessed in the ways purely physical phenomena can. But even non-measurable, non-reproducible phenomena can be observed and reported with care. I want to be part of those conversations and to learn what I can from those who have patiently followed alternative paths as healers.

I'm not a convert or a defector. I'm grateful for the many benefits of American medicine (though too few have access to them) and I need you, my kind and competent MD. I also think we need licensed tai-chi instructors, and massage therapists, and authentic faith healers; we need a wide range of people whose calling is healing, and who are trained observers and careful, caring guides who help others toward wholeness, integration, alignment, awareness, spiritual, physical, good mental health, and joy on the journey.

I don't believe venturing into non-Western medicine conflicts with my basic understanding of biology, anatomy, and physiology, or with my faith. It does, though, remind me of how the outer edges of all knowledge verge on mystery, and that the best way to live as we continue learning is, as Rabbi Abraham Heschel suggested, in "radical amazement."

My Two Minutes: What alternative or complementary approaches to medicine appeal to you? Which ones have you actually drawn upon in your practice?

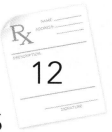

MONEY MATTERS

Disease is the biggest money maker in our economy.

—JOHN H. TOBE

Money may be the husk of many things but not the kernel. It brings you food, but not appetite; medicine, but not health.

—HENRIK IBSEN

I will remember that I do not treat a fever chart, a cancerous growth, but a sick human being, whose illness may affect the person's family and economic stability. My responsibility includes these related problems, if I am to care adequately for the sick.

—2019 VERSION OF THE HIPPOCRATIC OATH

Even though I have, by American standards, a fairly good health insurance plan, I put off visits to your office, or to my dentist, that might be advisable but don't seem urgent. I don't want to hand over the $35–$50 copay just to hear a dermatologist declare that the mole on my arm is "nothing" or to learn what I can easily read from WebMD or mayoclinic.org, or from conversations with friends who have had similar symptoms. I occasionally postpone filling prescriptions because it's less expensive to wait and see if my immune system will take care of the problem. These may be risky habits, but I know I'm not alone.

Health care is unnervingly expensive, even for those of us who are fairly healthy and have steady, if limited, incomes. Drugs are overpriced, and many of them are overprescribed. This is not your fault; you and other doctors I know do your best to minimize costs where you can by means of generic drugs, insurance codes, and at least pausing before prescribing when waiting might let a condition "clear up." I also know many patients come to you wanting prescriptions and go away disgruntled if they can't have them. They've watched the ads. We've all drunk the Kool-Aid. We're caught in a system that works primarily to the benefit of huge drug companies who make their billions from chronic conditions that require perpetual pills.

I'm sure you're well aware medical costs are the number one cause of bankruptcy in the US. Some sources report that two-thirds of bankruptcies are attributed to medical costs. *Healthcare Finance* reports that 56 percent of US adults attribute financial hardships to medical costs. While the Affordable Care Act helped many of us, neither the coverage nor the number of people covered was adequate. So here we still are—ranking near the bottom of industrialized countries in health, according to a 2018 article by Sally C. Pipes of the Pacific Research Institute, largely because our health care system has become so expensive, confusing, and disengaged from the daily decisions people make about food, drink, child care, and work stresses. That failure to serve basic human needs in the richest country in the world, however you spin it, is obscene.

I know some folks still vigorously maintain the fiction of having one of the best health care systems in the world, but statistics suggest that we're poorly fed, overmedicated, and suffering from preventable chronic diseases partly because of the system that claims to be helping us get well, if not stay well. Atul Gawande writes, "The soaring cost of health care has become the greatest threat to the long-term solvency of most advanced nations." This includes ours. Let's face it: you're stressed,

I'm stressed, and we don't have much time to talk about those stresses during our brief consultation.

When you urge me to take care of myself, I wonder how much time you think I have to go to the gym, or how much money I have for a gym membership. I wonder how much leisure most of your patients have for the kinds of self-care you wisely recommend. It takes some careful strategizing even to make sure I walk a few miles a few days a week. When I think of those who work longer hours, have more children, and have less discretionary income than I do, it's not surprising that sickness has become so normal. "Garden-variety" conditions you see in your office every day—obesity, fatigue, high blood pressure, persistent low-level coughs, and infections—must seem inconsequential now, so it must be easy to prescribe and move on rather than take time out of your own demanding days to lobby for more preventive medicine, help the AMA challenge food producers on pesticides, and track environmental toxins. Time is money. Most of us—you included—have to budget both carefully.

You and I don't talk about finances. I do that with the billing office. But I think it might help if we did acknowledge that money is one of the primary stressors and a health plan that doesn't consider this isn't very effective. Sentences that start with "You might want to . . ." often end with something I might indeed want to do, but can't afford: *You might want to get a massage once a month. Or see a skin-care specialist. Or go to the headache clinic. Or look into a retirement home for your mother.*

This statement from *The Locust Effect* struck me hard:

> The poor are the ones who can never afford to have any bad luck. They can't get an infection because they don't have access to any medicine. They can't get sick or miss their bus or get injured because they will lose their menial labor job if they don't show up for work. They can't misplace their pocket change because it's actually the only money they have left for food.

We veered uncomfortably close to this vortex when I was a kid. I remember my mother's home remedies not only as comforting throwbacks to an earlier time, but also as ways to avoid expensive trips to the doctor. I also remember that, even as a small child, I was somehow aware my weekly penicillin shots for nephritis were a stress on family resources.

Haugen and others (including the many who live in tents at the edges of freeways) have made me more acutely aware of the daily tradeoffs people who live right at the poverty line make. They see doctors only for the direst conditions, and often too late for effective treatment because it's too expensive. Most do take their children to doctors when the need is urgent, but many risk their jobs by sacrificing work hours to do so. David K. Shipler, another writer who has helped me see the link between poverty and health care with new eyes, connects even more dots. As he describes the predicament in which even ordinary, occasional illness leaves the working poor:

> On the surface, it seems odd that an interest rate can be determined by the condition of an apartment, which in turn can generate illness and medical bills, which may then translate into a poor credit rating, which limits the quality of an automobile that can be purchased, which jeopardizes a worker's reliability in getting to work, which limits promotions and restricts the wage, which confines a family to the dilapidated apartment. Such are the interlocking deficits of poverty, one reinforcing the other until an entire structure of want has been built.

Rereading those sentences reinforces my conviction that every health problem is a public health problem. Medicine, health care, and health maintenance are never separable from money. Even when, as in my insurance plan, a large percentage of the costs are covered, the costs are so high those remaining small percentages easily become daunting.

Those of us who can manage enough financial hurdles to get to your office still have to make our way through bureaucratic thickets that impose hidden costs along the way. Recently, I came in for a routine visit and ended up sliding my card into three different machines to pay at three different stations for three different procedures, two of which were arguably unnecessary. The operative word there is "routine." What has become routine is likely counted among "best practices," and you and others prescribe those routine procedures without much discussion of costs and benefits. Consigning the money conversation to people downstairs means you get to maintain the polite fiction that money somehow isn't an issue in our office visits. Bureaucracy hides and neutralizes and normalizes much that needs to be questioned. I'd like you to raise some of those questions from your corner of the building. I'll raise them from mine. Perhaps we could take our two minutes one of these times to talk tactics.

I don't like polite fictions. They're dangerous. Pretending a medical practice or procedure is somehow economically neutral is similar to pretending medicine is politically neutral. We both know we inhabit a system dominated by corporate interests that don't always work for my best interests or yours. Their primary obligation, as corporate orthodoxy goes, is to their stockholders. As not a few journalists and critics of Big Pharma have pointed out, sick people are a source of immense profit. This unsettling fact is underscored by another: "The pharmaceutical industry overall spends about twice as much on marketing and promotion as it does on research and development." Does this bother you? Or the fact that chronic disease is a source of steady income for investors?

I can simultaneously say I'm grateful for life-saving drugs and the scientists at their lab benches who produce them, and I'm also skeptical about pharmaceutical advertising. I've found other doubters more informed than I am who offer this kind of warning: "Most of all, immunize yourself from the drug companies' efforts to convince you that you desperately need their advertised products. If you really needed the product, it is unlikely that drug companies would be spending money on advertising. Remember, there aren't many ads for insulin on TV." I know doctors, and I know you're one of them, who share the skepticism, impatience, or moral qualms. I wonder if you'd share with me now and then two minutes' worth of reflection on how to stay resistant, resilient, and judicious and to keep a sense of direction about treatment options in the fog of influence peddling and propaganda.

I wonder what you ask yourself before you prescribe. I wonder when you have a chance to step back and ask questions about who determines "best practices" for prescribing medications or how the new and novel become normal, and then normative. Practicing medicine for profit, though you have to do it, does put you in a situation of inherent tension. You can't always do what you do on terms that make the best medical sense to you. You can't even make medical sense of what you observe without the benefit of training that is deeply embedded in a system funded and driven by corporate interests. Medical information, both to you and to us patients, is filtered. There are ways to bypass those filters, but they require time, intention, and sometimes courage. Do you have the courage to keep one foot outside the system you inhabit? I hope you do. If we both keep a critical eye on the way money shapes medicine, perhaps we can find the balance required to stay human and humane, and retain a sense of humor, and keep our eyes trained a little above the bottom line.

And yes, I know you can't change the system yourself. Even the physicians' associations to which you belong have limited political power relative to pharmaceutical lobbies and other large for-profit interests. But I think if we talked more frequently and freely about money in medicine, something might shift.

In the meantime, I hope and trust that you cling to the life-sustaining notion that medicine is a calling before it is a business—and that if it is a business, whose business you are minding, and for whose benefit, is a matter for vigorous moral discernment. The best visits I've had with you are those in which it becomes clear, as you explain or advise, that you love what you do. It is heartening to see that medicine has remained a passion and a vocation for you. We're in this together—partnered—and it seems good for both of us to keep alive the idea that the common good and "general welfare" of all the people around us opens a wider way to health.

My Two Minutes: How has money affected your approach to the work you do? How much do you have to concern yourself with medical practice as a business?

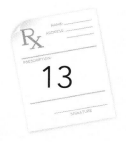

MUSIC MATTERS

> Music can be a powerful adjunct to the healing process. And music is one of the safest medicines you'll ever find. You can dose yourself as you please with no worries about toxic side effects.
> —ALLAN HAMILTON

> Music is not just music, it is medicine for the soul.
> —LIL WAYNE

ENOUGH ABOUT MONEY. LET'S talk about music. Unlike money, most of us can make music, listen to it, or at least hum a few bars from a favorite song that gives us a little pleasure and peace. One way or another, music is an affordable part of health care and one that deserves more acknowledgment in those two extra minutes we might have to talk about what helps me stay healthy.

I've been moved and motivated by the research that's happening in music and sound therapy. The kinds of healing music therapists can assist with cover an impressive range—from lessening the effects of dementia, to reducing asthma episodes or pain, to improving motor function for people with Parkinson's. They work in hospitals or meet with clients in studios where they compose, play, and sing together. They work with guitars, pianos, synthesizers, or even computers or smartphones that enable them and patients to listen to playlists that—sometimes with astonishing speed and specificity—redirect their energies, recharge their spirits, and relieve their pain. In his book *The Scalpel and the Soul*, neurosurgeon Allan Hamilton writes, "Music can be a powerful adjunct to the healing process. And music is one of the safest medicines you'll ever find. You can dose yourself as you please with no worries about toxic side effects." So if I "let music be my medicine," I might tap into a natural capacity for resilience that begins with a simple beat.

The ancient Greeks knew this. In case you didn't get enough medical history in school, consider Plato: "Harmony, which has motions akin to the revolutions of the Soul within us, was given by the Muses . . . as an auxiliary to the inner revolution of the Soul, when it has lost its harmony, to assist in restoring it to order and concord with itself." He and other ancients believed that music helped with catharsis and purification. Particular tones and instruments were prescribed for particular conditions. The value of those insights and the practices derived from them has been recognized by physicians, healers, musicians, and poets in succeeding generations. For instance, Francis Bacon, who wrote of the ancients, says, "The poets did well to conjoin music and medicine . . . because the office of medicine is but to tune the curious harp of man's body and reduce it to harmony."

That may be a somewhat oversimplified description of the "office of medicine," but it seems worth considering, and perhaps even entertaining it, as an objective to list among "healing outcomes." Imagine what might shift if you did! I think we have much to learn from those lyre-strumming Greeks, and from other cultures where music is a standard dimension of healing practice. Recent studies have shown that chants from various traditions provide beneficial effects on health and well-being.

During a difficult period in graduate school when I was living alone, suffering from debilitating depression and struggling to meet the ordinary requirements of daily life, I lay on the floor every evening and listened to Samuel Barber's "Adagio for Strings." Occasionally, I varied that ritual by playing two of the opening choruses in Brahms's *A German Requiem*. Neither is exactly upbeat and probably not for everyone; but for me, these pieces created a safe place for sadness and, over time, helped translate that sadness into a calmer, more reflective state of awareness in which something life-giving could begin to flourish.

As I began to emerge from that period of darkness and reclaim hope, I found myself strengthened and encouraged by two of Bach's gentlest, most lyrical choral works, *Bist du bei mir* ("If you are with me") and *Schafe können sicher weiden* ("Sheep may safely graze"). I was also, I might mention, energized and equipped for many days by Joni Mitchell and James Taylor and the Beatles—all of which no doubt dates me. You're younger than I am. Fill in your own playlist!

Music, then and now, offers me refuge from sorrow, confusion, and even physical pain. I remember getting through each childbirth with the help of Gilbert and Sullivan. The resonant sound of Tibetan bells has helped me through miserable afternoons in bed with the flu. So I take the claim that "music is medicine" quite literally.

Here's one more reason I do that: years ago, after having attended a drum circle at a retreat center where forty-some participants ended up in a spontaneous circle dance, I came home and wrote the following piece, "Beat." It began:

> The first thing we hear is a heartbeat. Crying babies, I'm told, can be quieted not only by being held close to a human heart, but even (though less cozily, to be sure) by setting a metronome or a ticking clock nearby. One of the earliest forms of play we engage in is to beat on anything in sight; every parent knows the sound of a rattle beating on crib bars or a wooden spoon on a pan. What we're doing, in our wise baby way, is tuning in to the rhythms of life with emphatic declarative trochees that assert our place in the world: "I'm here!" "I want!" "I can!"

Some cultures are better than ours at fostering a deep awareness that rhythms shape how we live and move. Rereading that piece, I am reminded of how music lightens my spirit and restores me. When I'm deeply fatigued, I lie down, listen to it, and take it into my body—not just into my ears, but also into my cells. It's very like drinking water when I'm thirsty or eating when I'm hungry. As Hoda Kotb put it, "A good song is like a good meal—I just want to inhale it and then share a bite with someone else." The sharing part is important: while music can enrich my solitude, it can also help me emerge from isolation or loneliness. That desire to "share a bite with someone else" nudges me toward resuming contact with people I love. It allows me to rise and walk. It's an instrument of healing. How can I encourage you to use it?

One way I can imagine your incorporating music into your medical practice is in the care and treatment of people with dementia. If you haven't seen *Alive Inside*, a documentary about the Music and Memory Project, do! In scene after scene, you see what happens when earphones are placed on people with advanced dementia. The music wakes people up who have been staring at the wall in apathetic isolation, and sometimes moves them to get up and dance. Some remember the words to songs and begin to sing. The brain cells that are gone don't regenerate, of course, but the parts of the brain that respond to music are galvanized into activity. Many volunteers in the hospice organization where I work participate in a Music and Memory program. As I age, I pray to be spared those particular mental afflictions, but I also imagine the music I listen to and love might somehow equip me to manage whatever effects of aging might come with resilience and grace. Maybe I should bring you a playlist of favorites to include in my medical record. They're already in my "Five Last Wishes."

When I sing, I am happier and healthier. Singing hymns with my mother was a fundamental part of my spiritual education. The week after she died, I awoke three mornings in a row with one of her favorite hymns playing in my head. Those hymns helped me through my grief and recognize how much life she had imparted. They also helped me reclaim my own life without her. Singing with my children saw us through some of the most challenging chapters of family life; as they learned to harmonize by singing rounds, I believe they came into deeper harmony with each other.

Music saw my generation through the televised horrors of Vietnam, and I have seen since then how generations of students have sought refuge in music from the deep stresses of apocalyptic threats. One teaching doctor I worked with had a music night with students every month or two. Imagine singing as part of medical education! Imagine being a doctor who sings! Imagine prescribing drumming practice for the weak of heart.

Making music has come to seem more urgent to me of late as the morning news becomes more dire and awareness of new kinds and a new scale of suffering has impinged more frequently on my consciousness. I've begun flute lessons again, knowing I'll likely never do more than play simple duets with my husband at the piano, because I find the sound of the flute consoling and centering. When I'm ill, I would love for you to be a doctor who paid some attention to how music (and which music) might help.

You wouldn't be alone if you did. Three doctors who are widely revered—Oliver Sacks, Atul Gawande, and Danielle Ofri—bring imaginative and eclectic approaches to clinical practice. They attest to the value of music in the clinic, the hospital, and even the surgical theater, where Gawande works to an energizing background of indie music. Sacks's book *Musicophilia* makes accessible a surprising range of research about music and the brain. He writes about diagnosable conditions that directly correlate to how the brain processes music. And Ofri describes emotions as the "continuous musical line of our minds, the unstoppable humming."

It's not only within us, but also all around us. Paying attention to the musicality of birdsong, and wind, and even traffic might provide valuable information about how our internal and external soundscapes affect both emotional and physiological processes. Maybe, if you do more of this for yourself, you'll find yourself prescribing music. Or at least occasionally sharing it in ways that might help us both. As poet Richard Wilbur put it, to see:

In all bodies the beat of spirit,
Not merely in the *tout en l'air*
Or double pike with layout

But in the strong,
Shouldering gait of the legless man,
The calm walk of the blind young woman
Whose cane touches the curbstone.

It may be that what the stethoscope tells you goes beyond heart rate and rhythm and how well valves are working. If you listen in, maybe it will remind you, every time, to notice the "beat of spirit" in the person whose health depends, at least in part, on a distant drummer.

My Two Minutes: What music do you listen to? What music helps you when you're tired or sick or sad?

LIFE IMITATES ART

The skills I learned studying fine arts in college are invaluable to me now as a physician.
—Jaclyn Gurwin, MD

If I do not violate this oath, may I enjoy life and art.
—2019 Version of the Hippocratic Oath

While we're humming our way to health, let's also talk about how a little paint might change a life. Medical schools may not have been doing it when you were enrolled, but dozens of them have begun to require some instruction in visual art over the past few years. Some of them offer whole semester courses that include trips to museums and conversations about how art can teach students to see in ways that may make them more astute diagnosticians. Some of the schools just bring in a few speakers with pictures on PowerPoint. Some offer opportunities for informal studio art instruction. All of them are taking at least a few steps to acknowledge the role of the arts in healing. Doesn't this make you want to hasten back to your alma mater and listen in? Or go to one of the conferences or Continuing Medical Education seminars where they're doing the same thing? I've had a chance to do this a few times and I can tell you, it's exhilarating to watch a roomful of doctors gazing at a painting by Munch and musing on the insights it offers about pain or anxiety or altered states or mental disorder.

At Penn State Medical School, Dr. Michael Flanagan makes exciting claims about a course he teaches, focused largely on Monet and Van Gogh, that opens up conversations about mental illness and cognitive bias. He writes: "It's protecting and maintaining students' empathy, so that by the time they go off to practice medicine, they're still empathetic individuals." Since recent studies have shown— insofar as it's measurable—that students' empathy decreases significantly by the time the pressures of the third year set in (and who knows how decreased it is by the twelfth year of medical practice?) this offset is no small achievement.

There are other ways art and medicine can intersect even for you, entrenched as you are in an established practice. Consider this story and see if it offers some possibilities. I had an unusual chance, during the period when my aforementioned migraines were worst, to work with a doctor who made me be the artist. He handed me a box of crayons and a sheet of drawing paper, and asked me, as I believe I mentioned above, to draw an image of myself with a migraine. After a moment's hesitation, during which I had to set aside my inhibitions about drawing—not one of my finer skills—I sketched an image of a figure surrounded by bright yellow with streaks of red, encased in what looked like a black cocoon. I drew a couple of other images in the course of our short session, but that figure remains in my mind, partly because I recognized in it, when I put down the crayons, something strikingly true to my experience of migraine—enclosure to the point of claustrophobia, but also a sensation of unbearable brightness in the presence of any direct light. The doctor took the time—and it didn't require much—to ask me a few salient questions about what I'd drawn. It was like reflecting on dream images—something I've also found valuable. A cocoon, I remember observing, is a place where growth and transformation are taking place. The image struck me at the time as curiously hopeful: the experience of migraine might actually offer me some occasion for enhanced awareness, learning, unfolding new layers of consciousness. In retrospect, I believe it did. And I believe the time spent that day, taken from a doctor's busy schedule, changed the nature of my participation in healing a long-standing affliction that has ebbed into very minor and infrequent headaches. Nevertheless, the vivid memory of pain has helped me empathize with others who suffer.

That doctor, no doubt because he also worked as a therapist, had arranged a work life that allowed for the time it took to do exploratory art work. I know you can't do that in the same way, or perhaps at all, but I bet it wouldn't take more than two extra minutes to explain to me, or some other patient, what might happen if they went home and spent a little time drawing. And then to look at a drawing together on the next visit. What do you think? If you tell me to, I'll dig out my crayons and bring them.

I mentioned earlier the exhibit of "migraine art" I saw some time after the day of the cocoon drawing. I entered the exhibit hesitantly, wondering if the images might in fact trigger a headache of the sort they represented. Some were violent—a giant screw driven into the occipital area of a person's skull; twisted faces reminiscent of Munch's "The Scream"; jagged lightning bolts aimed at head and neck, and a number of abstract pieces that suggested electrical storms or a tangle of underwater vegetation. I wasn't triggered; I was fascinated. I realized how various the experience of pain is, and how, as with many diagnoses, a single term, "migraine," can cover a range of experiences. The same, of course, is true for cancer or flu or Parkinson's or multiple sclerosis. In every body disease is a new event— hence my insistence that each of us is a "special case."

A sizeable gallery of art by patients and caregivers, including doctors and nurses, is available on the internet. A host of illnesses and disabilities are represented. Take a look, for instance, at Angela Canada Hopkins's wildly colorful "Cancer Cell No. 19," or at Tim Lowly's stirring paintings of his daughter Temma, who has cerebral palsy with spastic quadriplegia. He calls her "a great and utterly innocent mystery," and helps us see her that way. Look at Alice Neel's Works Progress Administration portraits of the poor in Spanish Harlem who suffered from tuberculosis. Altogether, looking at art by and about people dealing with illness, injury, disability, or dying is both inspiring and convincing: art helps heal, even when it doesn't cure. Sometimes it points a way to cure. At the very least, art brings people who are suffering out of isolation into community. Art in hospitals, art in clinics and doctors' offices, and opportunities for patients to make and share art that communicates something unique about their conditions all seem to me signs of life and hope in the very health care system I've been critiquing. Professionals who work to bring arts and medicine together have determined that artwork in patient rooms promotes healing, relieves patients' pain and stress, and increases their overall well-being.

Of course, not all art related to medicine and illness promotes well-being. Movies and TV series like *ER*, *Scrubs*, and *Grey's Anatomy* have romanticized, sensationalized, oversimplified, and otherwise distorted medical practice, and probably patients' expectations of the magic you may be able to work (or if not, why not?). I recognize that I'm susceptible, along with the rest of the vast viewing audience, to those distortions; I've squandered evening hours watching sexy young people in white coats dash around hospital corridors and peer into open chest cavities in the OR, and I'm sure those images leave an imprint somewhere in my reptilian brain, against which I measure the pedestrian realities of hospital life when I see it. I'm sure they affect my notions about medical authority, the power of drugs and technology. They also reinforce some of my inhibitions about talking with people in white coats (this lengthy letter notwithstanding!), and a general feeling of powerlessness as a patient. In those shows, decisions are made behind closed doors. Patients generally don't have much access. Ethics violations infuse plotlines enough to make some of us feel nervous about what happens behind those closed doors. And institutional practices that might deserve to be questioned or held up for critical scrutiny are normalized—schedules

that leave practitioners sleep-deprived, communication pro-
tocols that disempower nurses, and dramatic interventions
that are far more rare in reality than they're made to look.

There are mirrors all around us—not only in movies,
but also in pop-up ads and full-page magazine spreads and
on billboards—that distort notions of the doctor-patient
relationship, sickness and health, childbirth, disability, death
and dying. It's a challenge to "keep it real." Yet despite these
distortions, art offers life-giving possibilities. You could help
me, and the rest of us languishing in the waiting room, to
sustain that well-being in some pretty simple ways.

I bet you could afford to experiment with some wall
space—maybe take down the posters of the muscular
system or the color-coordinated motel-room prints and
put up a painting by a woman with breast cancer or a
drawing by a child with asthma. I would love to see a
little rotating art gallery in your office; it might give me
a sense of how you see and who you are and who are my
fellow patients—those people quietly sniffling and reading magazines in the reception area. I also want to assure
you that if you invited me to draw something about my
current complaints, however inexpert, you might (and I
might) find out something that would otherwise escape
our notice. These days I might, if I were to paint my pain,
venture into the kind of abstract expressionism that could

give shape and color to the anxieties I carry, or to what an irritable bowel or arthritic knee feels like. My brave artist friend whose Parkinson's is progressing might post a series of shaky images that offer a poignant but interesting record of that progression. Maybe my nephew would post one of his edgy cartoons about what it feels like to drip through a common cold with a red nose, nausea, and a teacher who thinks a cold is an excuse slackers make.

In other words, our conversation, no matter what the "presenting complaint," might benefit from at least a passing allusion to art, now and then, not only for its interest value, since you know I'm interested, but also because it might make you an even better doctor. I'm not, please note, suggesting you take up painting in your spare time or muddy those clean fingers throwing pots (though neither would be a bad use of your—um—*many* leisure hours). What I am suggesting is that making some place for art in your life or reminding me of the life-giving importance of it in mine in the few brief shining moments we share, might yield surprising results.

My Two Minutes: What one or two works of art would you visit if you could? When have you been powerfully affected by a statue, painting, play, or film?

I Am Made from This Earth

We know ourselves to be made from this earth.
We know this earth is made from our bodies.
For we see ourselves. And we are nature.
We are nature seeing nature. We are nature
with a concept of nature. Nature weeping.
Nature speaking of nature to nature.

—Susan Griffin

I will protect the environment which sustains us,
in the knowledge that the continuing health of
ourselves and our societies is dependent on a
healthy planet.

—2019 Version of the Hippocratic Oath

ALONG WITH OTHER ENGLISH majors and those some might call poetry nerds, I have laughed over John Donne's rhapsodic words in "To His Mistress Going to Bed": "Oh, my America! My new-found-land!" Exploring the topography of her body, he makes a bawdy point, but also one I've found myself reflecting on in idle moments, and again when, tracking the geography of persistent, annoying aches and itches—my body as I imagine it, with its inaccessible, unexplored areas, harbors undiscovered territory.

I find the fact that we are composed primarily of six elements (oxygen, carbon, hydrogen, nitrogen, calcium, and phosphorus, a list I once memorized with awe) both humbling and exhilarating. The chemicals we're made of I learned, are common and relatively cheap, but also awe-inspiring in their origins. "The atoms of our bodies," Neil de Grasse Tyson writes, "are traceable to stars that manufactured them in their cores and exploded these enriched ingredients across our galaxy, billions of years ago." That makes you, me—everyone—biologically connected to every other living thing in the world. Everyone out there in the waiting room. Everyone being born and dying. Everyone being wheeled around in that hospital where you make your morning rounds. We are chemically connected to all molecules on Earth. And we are atomically connected to all atoms in the universe. We are literally stardust. And so is the dust that accumulates under the sofa along with lost hair pins, missing puzzle pieces, and dead insects—also stardust—all of it. When I think about that fact, I remain amazed. I hope after a day of peering at bodies, you can still be amazed too. I hope you get whatever you need from patients, family, colleagues, friends, reflection, or reading to sustain your awe.

Dust is important in my religious tradition. At the beginning of Lent when I hear the familiar words, "Remember that you are dust," I think of how earthy some of Jesus's healing encounters were: he spat in the dirt, made a mud paste, and smeared it on the eyes of the blind man. He walked right into the stink of the dead man Lazarus's rotting body to bring him back to a life of desert sun and his sisters' food. And, of course, Jesus was born in a feeding trough. Something in all those stories of incarnation and healing keeps reminding us that we are dust.

As the climate crisis turns mud into dust and parches the topsoil, public awareness of how we affect the environment and how the environment affects us seems to be growing, along with the fears that come with that awareness. I think often about the fact that what happens to the earth happens to our bodies. "A nation that destroys its soil destroys itself," Franklin Roosevelt presciently warned. And elsewhere he reminded us, "Forests are the 'lungs' of our land, purifying the air and giving fresh strength to our people."

My concerns about strip mining, soil depletion, plastic in the oceans, the effects of fracking on water quality, and the demise of bees are not separable from my concerns about my own health. As Wendell Berry wrote in a chapter called "The Body and the Earth," "To be healed we must come with all the other creatures to the feast of Creation." With them—not on them, or hanging their heads on walls, or draping ourselves in their skins, or dangling charms made of their tusks, but recognizing the common needs, and dependencies, and dangers that link us.

When I come to you, it is with some hope that you, too, see health and healing through a wide-angle lens—that you connect the dots, every time you look at my body—at any body—that link public "resource" policies to individual health concerns. I'd love to be assured that you care about water quality, for instance, perhaps enough to advise me knowledgeably about how to shop for the most effective water filters or how to hold the local water board accountable for water quality. I'd like to know which pollutants to be concerned about, where factory runoff is likely to leave coliform bacteria in the soil, what nearby industrial processes (or, indeed, as has happened, hospitals) are quietly disposing harmful substances upstream, what detergents and fertilizers are affecting marine habitats, as well as those of us who swim in those habitats or eat those marine animals. I'd like the medicine I count on for help to live right next door to environmental science.

I'd like to know that you concern yourself with local efforts to create and maintain green spaces, not only as beautiful places for retreat from the noise and haste of urban life, but also because they are crucial to life and health. That they are has been well documented, though not, apparently, well enough to change the design of concrete-block schools, prisons, and even healing facilities. According to Richard Louv, "Time in nature is not leisure time; it's an essential investment in our children's health." (And also, by the way, in our own.) He cites studies that show that even putting a plant in a hospital room helps people heal more quickly. Maybe a plant in your office would go a long way to offset institutional sterility with a little vibrant hospitality.

The Lakota believe that "Man's heart away from nature becomes hard." Like so many body metaphors, this one seems to point to medical fact: hardened arteries and damaged hearts come from an industrialized diet of processed food transported long distances by fossil fuels, laced with preservatives, packaged in plastic, stripped of many nutrients, stuffed with chemical additives. Away from nature we get stiff necks and sore eyes and wrists sitting at computers, often in ergonomically awkward positions, ignoring body signals, deprived of natural light, wind, and plant life many hours a day. We become *high strung* or *strung out* or *tightly wound* when our muscles are contracted for too long without the release of free movement, bending, running, stretching. We become *shallow* as our polluted lungs make it harder for us to breathe deeply, and deforestation destroys the lungs of this planet. We are *scattered* and unfocused by chronic diffusion of our energies—as Eliot put it, "distracted from distraction by distraction." I'd like you to remember where our sources of healing lie and to help keep me and others alert to when we are moving "our hearts away from nature."

Our bodies, and the earth, suffer from disrupted cycles, depletion, overuse, misuse, colonization, exploitation, extraction, crowding, and various other kinds of abuse. Yet I believe even in the midst of all that, some hope may be claimed. As Vance Havner puts it, "God uses broken things. It takes broken soil to produce a crop, broken clouds to give rain, broken grain to give bread." These assailed and impaired and broken bodies—our flesh and bones and the planet's soil and oceans—are also resilient in "fearful and wonderful" ways, infused and alive with the Spirit that dwells in and moves through and among us like wind. I think our conversations about health need to keep this truth alive—that we are like the earth, that the earth mirrors us, that we are made of it, that it is our teacher, that it is our home.

Your office is a place where some of this cultural distancing could be named and healed. I'd like us to remind each other occasionally that whatever the "presenting complaint" may be, it mirrors something in the larger world that needs to be addressed. We carry messages for one another in our bodies. You are one of those appointed to read those messages and help interpret them. I hope you continue connecting the dots and helping me connect them. It's our job on this journey to keep each other accountable and active. Your activism and mine are part of the healing work we do together. Let's do it together. Help me to help you heal.

My Two Minutes: How do your concerns about the environment (air pollution, waste disposal, climate change, loss of biodiversity, etc.) shape your approach to medical work?

QUESTIONS I'D LIKE MY DOCTOR TO ASK

Dear Patient,

The answers to these questions are optional, but may help me help you. Unless you arrived awfully early, you won't have time to answer them all while you're in the waiting room, but look them over and see which ones might matter most to you. Perhaps we can at least begin a conversation about dimensions of health care that will widen our focus and help healing happen.

WITH RESPECT FROM
A DOCTOR WHO LOVES TO
KEEP LEARNING

1. How is the medical condition you've come to consult me about affecting your daily life, relationships, feelings about yourself?

2. In what ways does coming to see me make you apprehensive? How can I help make our visit more comfortable?

3. How do you feel your case may be a little different from others' with a similar condition?

4. Is there anything in particular that bothers you about the way medical people or people in general speak about your condition? Are there particular words that trigger you in some way?

5. What might inspire you to participate in your own healing by changing habits or attitudes?

6. Do you think of yourself as a "fighter"? If not, how might you describe how you are motivated to take action to make your life better?

7. Choose the verb you think best completes this sentence: "I am a person who _____."

8. Aside from what tastes good, what three or four foods most make you feel satisfied that you've given your body something good and life-giving?

9. Do you ever rely on a "higher power" to help you care for your health and well-being? What spiritual practices help you?

10. What fears do you experience when you think about your health? How do you cope with those fears? How can I help you cope with them?

11. When you think about your health in the long term, what helps you imagine your own aging and dying with clarity and equanimity? Have you found helpful ways to prepare for the next stages of your life?

12. Have you ever consulted a practitioner of alternative or "complementary" medicine (naturopath, acupuncturist, chiropractor, hypnotherapist, herbalist, Ayurvedic practitioner, energy healer, medical intuitive, etc.)? Have they helped you? Would you like to talk about ways to integrate the work you do with them and the work we do here?

13. Would you like to make time to talk about how money concerns affect your medical decision-making?

14. What kind of music do you find healing? Would you like some guidance in ways to make music part of your health care?

15. How do stories, films, art, crafts, and creative work help you? Would you like some suggestions about how to integrate them into your healing or long-term health maintenance?

16. How do you think your present condition relates to the health of the soil, water, and air, to the life of animals and plants, to public health concerns? Would you like to learn more about organizations that are concerned with care of the food system? Of earth's ecosystems and species?

A Brief Guide to Resources

One of the best resources available for people interested in thoughtful, wide-ranging approaches to medical care, health, and healing is the Literature Arts Medicine Database (http://medhum.med.nyu.edu), a website that posts brief reviews of literature, films, and artworks related to medicine. The "key word" search function makes it easy to find material related to a particular illness or issue in medical care.

Many documentaries about medicine, health, and healing are readily available. Helpful annotated lists may be found at https://www.mphonline.org/best-public-health-documentaries/ and https://www.syberscribe.com.au/blog/12-powerful-medical-documentaries-watch/.

A few fine TED talks on medicine, illness, health, and healing are listed here: https://www

.topmastersinhealthcare.com/15-inspiring-ted-talks-on
-health-and-medicine/.

Here is a short (and by no means comprehensive) list
of ten contemporary doctor authors whose reflections on
medicine I have found particularly helpful:

Rita Charon	Danielle Ofri
Nawal El Saadawi	Oliver Sacks
Atul Gawande	Rachel Naomi Remen
Paul Kalanithi	Abraham Verghese
Siddhartha Mukherjee	Brian Volck

Here is a short (also by no means comprehensive)
list of **patient authors** whose works I find especially
illuminating:

Chana Bloch (poetry)	Nancy Mairs (essays/ memoir)
Lucille Clifton (poetry)	
Cortney Davis (poetry/ memoir)	Adam Mars-Jones (fiction/memoir)
Karen Fiser (poetry)	Reynolds Price (memoir)
Susanna Kaysen (memoir)	Floyd Skloot (memoir)
	Lauren Slater (memoir)

FOR MY DOCTOR:
A COUNTER-QUESTIONNAIRE

You're about to see me and I'm about to see you. I understand you need information about me in order to help me. Therefore, these are my interview questions. They'll help me know on what terms we may "partner" in working for health and healing.

1. How do you think about the difference between "curing" and "healing"?

2. What do you do to minimize patients' embarrassment or to avoid humiliation during a physical exam?

3. Studies show that compassion or empathy for patients starts eroding by the third year of medical school. What do you do to sustain compassion

and empathy for and interest in patients—even those suffering from conditions you've seen many times?

4. What have you learned about how to translate effectively, not only from English to another language, but also from medicalese to common English without "dumbing down"? What "trigger" words have you learned to avoid? What has your work taught you about the importance of the language you use? What listening skills have you developed?

5. What are your alternatives to the militarized language that has become so common in medicine: *fighting disease, aggressive measures, bombardment, targeting*, etc.? How important is it to you that medicine demilitarize its language?

6. How do you stay focused on *who* I am, as well as *what* is wrong with me? On the life context in which I became ill or injured, as well as on the illness or injury itself?

7. How much did you learn about nutrition and food production when you were in med school? How does that awareness come into your assessment of

health or illness, and your decisions about prevention and treatment?

8. How do you honor patients' commitment to their own faith traditions or spiritual practices? Are you open to addressing the faith factor as you work with patients?

9. How much do you focus on prevention rather than just cure?

10. How do you help patients who are afraid?

11. How do you help patients who are nearing death? How do you determine when further treatment is "futile"? How do you help patients die with dignity?

12. What medical traditions and practices, other than conventional Western-European/American medical training, have you taken time to learn about (e.g., herbal medicine, Ayurvedic medicine, energy medicine, naturopathy, homeopathy, meditation, etc.)? How do you integrate any of these into your work with patients? If you don't, how do you support patients who pursue any of these avenues of healing?

13. Do you talk with patients about the financial cost of treatment or do you leave that to the office staff? How do you help patients navigate the complexities of the insurance system, or at least address their anxieties about doing so? Are you politically active in helping bring about more equitable and universal access to health care?

14. How do you embrace the value of art, music, story, or poetry in healing and health? For instance, do you ever "prescribe" music? Or make visual art a part of your work environment?

15. How do you address the larger contexts of illness—public health, environmental degradation, allergens, soil depletion, etc.—as you talk with patients about what makes them sick? What do you do to support environmental causes?

16. What questions do you ask yourself to keep growing and owning your edge?

Notes

INTRODUCTION

The time primary-care physicians have to spend with each patient is . . .

"Amount of Time US Primary Care Physicians Spent with Each Patient as of 2018," Statista, released April 2018, https://tinyurl.com/tpp7nxy. On frequency of interruptions, see Bruce Y. Lee, "11 Seconds: How Long Your Doctor Listens before Interrupting You," *Forbes*, July 22, 2018, https://tinyurl.com/tpll59w.

CHAPTER 1

"Shame can be exacerbated or even incited by physicians . . .

Luna Dolezal, "The Phenomenology of Shame in the Clinical Encounter," *Medicine, Health Care, and Philosophy* 18, no. 4 (November 2015): 567.

"I will remember that there is art to medicine as well as science . . ."

Wikipedia chronicles a short history of versions of the Hippocratic Oath, including the 2019 version from which this comes. Wikipedia, s.v., "Hippocratic Oath," last modified February

14, 2020, 7:22 (UTC), https://tinyurl.com/qm67386. See also Vanessa Bates Ramirez, "Why Medicine Needs a New Hippocratic Oath—and What It Should Be," SingularityHub, https://tinyurl.com/r6w33lz.

"Many Americans say they would rather live in pain than visit their doctor."

"Study Reveals Patient-Doctor Disconnect on Healthy Living," Business Wire, February 16, 2010, https://tinyurl.com/vh7tk7v.

. . . most of us "have grown up feeling alienated in our bodies, embarrassed or ashamed of them, not at home in our physical selves."

Lucy H. Pearce, *Medicine Woman: Reclaiming the Soul of Healing* (Cork, Ireland: Womancraft Publishing, 2018), 21.

". . . [We] have internalized the message that there's something wrong with us, rather than there is something wrong."

Pearce, *Medicine Woman*, 21.

"We're always trotting out some story of a ninety-seven-year-old who runs marathons . . ."

Atul Gawande, *Being Mortal: Medicine and What Matters in the End* (New York: Metropolitan Books, 2017), 28.

". . . specific instruction and evaluation . . ."

Liaison Committee on Medical Education, *Functions and Structure of a Medical School* (Washington, DC: Liaison Committee on Medical Education, 1998), as cited in Gregory Makoul, "Communication Skills Education in Medical School and Beyond," *JAMA* 289, no. 1 (January 2003): 93, https://doi.org/10.1001/jama.289.1.93.

"'Go ahead and push once for me,' Dr. Oliver said."
Ree Drummond, *The Pioneer Woman: Black Heels to Tractor Wheels—A Love Story* (New York: William Morrow Paperbacks, 2012), 294.

"The purpose was to help us become more thoughtful and meticulous observers . . ."
Dhruv Khullar, MD, "What Doctors Can Learn from Looking at Art," *New York Times*, December 22, 2016, https://tinyurl.com/tytt5a7.

"an experience of a very high order."
Roberto Gerhard, *Gerhard on Music: Selected Writings*, ed. Meirion Bowen (New York: Routledge, 2019), 13 and 29.

CHAPTER 2

"True patient-centered care requires providers and practices to forge strong partnerships with patients and families."
"Partnering with Patients to Improve Quality, Safety, and the Patient Experience," Agency for Healthcare Research and Quality (May 2016): 1, https://tinyurl.com/rguw87m.

"It became rather difficult . . ."
Pamela N. Munster, *Twisting Fate: My Journey with BRCA—from Breast Cancer Doctor to Patient and Back* (New York: The Experiment, 2018), 73–74.

. . . that fine-tuning food practices needs to be part of my health plan.
One of several useful lists of valuable documentaries about food and health may be found at *https://greenpress.co/blogs/news/78588102-top-10-health-food-documentaries.*

"I feared I was losing sight of the singular importance of human relationship . . ."

Paul Kalanithi, *When Breath Becomes Air* (New York: Random House, 2016), 86.

CHAPTER 3

Here's an exquisite poem titled "Stranded" about post-surgery pain by Karen Fiser . . .

Karen Fiser, "Stranded," in *Words Like Fate and Pain* (Cambridge, MA: Zoland Books, 1992), 10.

It makes you self-aware in new ways—of your raw sentience and your mortality.

Fiser's first collection of poems is *Words Like Fate and Pain*. The message of its title and text throughout the remarkable collection is that words matter. They change the memory and meaning of pain. They reframe what fate delivers.

. . . Linda Pastan, imagines herself crouching . . .

Linda Pastan, "Migraine," in *An Early Afterlife: Poems* (New York: W. W. Norton, 1995), 68.

Alexandre Arnau, another migraine sufferer, writes of . . .

Alexandre Arnau, "Migraine," submitted August 16, 2005, https://tinyurl.com/stuj5fg.

A third poet, Katherine Larson, describes migraine as a "dark anchor" lodged behind the eyes.

Katherine Larson, "Love at Thirty-Two Degrees," Poetry Foundation, accessed October 19, 2018, https://tinyurl.com/rkyqetp. This poem was also printed in the March 2006 issue of *Poetry Magazine*.

And another, Cathy Song, recounts her exploration of pain with the precision of a scientific observer.

Cathy Song, "Youngest Daughter," Poetry Foundation, accessed October 20, 2018, https://tinyurl.com/w5qq2ul. This poem was originally printed in Cathy Song's *The Picture Bride* (New Haven, CT: Yale University Press, 1983).

CHAPTER 4

"Words can strengthen the weak . . ."

Abhijit Naskar, *Time to Save Medicine* (Seattle: Amazon Publishing Company, 2018), 11.

"Words, after speech, reach . . ."

T. S. Eliot, "Burnt Norton," *Four Quartets* (Boston: Mariner Books, 1968), 19.

"Learning medicine," Daniel Kahneman wrote, "consists in part of learning the language of medicine."

Daniel Kahneman, *Thinking, Fast and Slow* (New York: Farrar, Straus and Giroux, 2013), 3.

He said if he could explain it in three minutes, it wouldn't be worth a Nobel Prize.

Lee Dye, "Nobel Physicist R. P. Feynman of Caltech Dies," *Los Angeles Times*, February 16, 1988, https://tinyurl.com/s8qcbvq.

Aurora Levins Morales, writing about the culture and politics of medicine . . .

Aurora Levins Morales, *Medicine Stories: History, Culture and the Politics of Integrity* (Cambridge, MA: South End Press, 1998), 37.

Maybe you have read Broyard's book . . .
> Anatole Broyard, *Intoxicated by My Illness and Other Writings on Life and Death* (New York: Ballantine Books, 1992), 18.

One is to "introduce unfamiliar material" to patients . . .
> Vyjeyanthi S. Periyakoil, MD, "Using Metaphors in Medicine," Stanford School of Medicine: Palliative Care, January 2016, https://tinyurl.com/vxbxs7y.

". . . Lacking the language to discuss mortality is the ultimate way of erasing it."
> Sunita Puri, *That Good Night: Life and Medicine in the Eleventh Hour* (New York: Viking, 2019), 93.

. . . and the final lines of Jane Kenyon's exquisite poem . . .
> Jane Kenyon, "Let Evening Come," in *Collected Poems* (Saint Paul, MN: Graywolf, 2005), 213.

In Abraham Verghese's beautiful novel about coming of age into a life in medicine . . .
> Abraham Verghese, *Cutting for Stone* (New York: Vintage, 2010), 520.

Joyce Sequichie Hilfer restores words to their rightful place among instruments of healing and human flourishing.
> Joyce Sequichie Hifler, *A Cherokee Feast of Days: Daily Meditations* (Tulsa, OK: Council Oak Books, 1992), 264.

CHAPTER 5

"In Beyond AIDS: A Journey into Healing . . ."
> Anne Hunsaker Hawkins, *Reconstructing Illness: Studies in Pathography* (West Lafayette, IN: Purdue University Press, 1998), 71.

Medical discourse is replete with the language of war . . .
>   Abraham Fuks, "The Military Metaphors of Modern Medicine," Semantic Scholar, accessed February 20, 2019, https://tinyurl.com/w6gcyet.

I think of the poignant question Dhruv Khullar raised in another piece about military metaphors in medicine . . .
>   Dhruv Khullar, "The Trouble with Medicine's Metaphors," *The Atlantic*, Aug. 7, 2014, https://tinyurl.com/wmp7lw3.

People telling you to 'keep fighting' when you're feeling weak . . .
>   "Battling, Brave or Victim: Why the Language of Cancer Matters," Breast Cancer Now, January 29, 2016, https://tinyurl.com/razt3ov.

CHAPTER 6

"I know that I am not a category."
>   R. Buckminster Fuller, *I Seem to Be a Verb* (Berkeley, CA: Gingko Press, 2015).

". . . endure their going hence, even as their coming hither."
>   William Shakespeare, *King Lear*, Act 5, Scene 2, https://tinyurl.com/tst2llc.

Hindu texts teach . . .
>   "Mahārāja Nimi Meets the Nine Yogendras," Śrīmad-Bhāgavatam, accessed February 9, 2020, https://tinyurl.com/um3qglo.

CHAPTER 7

"Real healthcare occurs outside of the doctor's office and hospitals"
Emmanuel Fombu, *The Future of Healthcare: Humans and Machines Partnering for Better Outcomes* (Athena Books, 2018), 229.

"Don't eat anything with more than five ingredients, or ingredients you can't pronounce."
Michael Pollan, as cited in Daniel J. DeNoon, "7 Rules for Eating," WebMD, March 23, 2009, https://tinyurl.com/tzj3fpy.

"The Association of American Medical Colleges (AAMC) has recently declined to incorporate nutrition . . ."
Kelly M. Adams, W. Scott Butsch, and Martin Kohlmeier, "The State of Nutrition Education at US Medical Schools," *Journal of Biomedical Education* 2015 (August 2015): 2, http://dx.doi.org/10.1155/2015/357627.

". . . Don't eat anything that won't eventually rot."
Pollan, "7 Rules for Eating."

Maybe you've read the Center for Accountability in Science's recent report about the state of food and drug research.
"Industry-Funded Research," Center for Accountability in Science, accessed December 26, 2019, https://tinyurl.com/syvjeju.

"Tasking the government agency that manages America's food production . . ."
Alexandra Sifferlin, "Here's What 10 Experts Think of the Government's New Diet Advice, *Time Magazine*, Jan. 7, 2016, https://tinyurl.com/rpf7hxj.

In 2016, a physicians committee at Grady Hospital in Atlanta, Georgia, sponsored three billboard ads challenging the hospital to go fast food free . . .

"Three Billboards Confront McDonald's at Grady Hospital," Physicians Committee for Responsible Medicine, May 10, 2016, https://tinyurl.com/qocaja9.

. . . the distressing reasons why Washington has not yet successfully curtailed the power of big food corporations . . .

Neal Barnard, MD, "Five Takeaways on the White House and Big Food," Physicians Committee for Responsible Medicine, October 7, 2016, https://tinyurl.com/udnmt4l.

CHAPTER 8

"Prayer . . . offers many of the same health and stress-relief benefits as meditation."

Rick Warren, Daniel Amen, and Mark Hymen, *The Daniel Plan: 40 Days to a Healthier Life* (Grand Rapids, MI: Zondervan, 2013).

"Not to employ prayer with my patients was the equivalent of deliberately withholding a potent drug or surgical procedure."

Larry Dossey, *Healing Words: The Power of Prayer and the Practice of Medicine* (New York: HarperOne, 1995), xviii.

One article posted on WebMD, however, claims that research focusing on the power of prayer in healing has nearly doubled over the past twenty years.

Jeanie Lerche Davis, "Can Prayer Heal?" WebMD, March 26, 2004, https://tinyurl.com/w7lzksg.

"Holiness is simply being connected to our Source."

Richard Rohr, "A School of Love," Center for Action and Contemplation, June 23, 2019, https://tinyurl.com/uteotjt.

None of us knows exactly how prayer "works" . . .
> Some progress has been made in understanding particle "entanglement," though questions about how it works remain unanswered. For some information on this, please see: Tia Ghose, "Entangled Particles Reveal Even Spookier Action Than Thought," Live Science, September 13, 2016, https://tinyurl.com/wsf7o6u.

". . . certain spiritual beliefs and the practice of prayer are associated with improved coping and better health outcomes."
> Marek Jantos and Hosen Kiat, "Prayer as Medicine: How Much Have We Learned?" *Medical Journal of Australia* 186, no. 10 (May 2007): S51, doi: 10.5694/j.1326-5377.2007.tb01041.x.

"Most studies have shown that religious involvement and spirituality are associated with better health outcomes . . ."
> E. Mohandas, MD, "Neurobiology of Spirituality," *Mens Sana Monogr* 6, no.1 (January–December 2008): 63–80, https://dx.doi.org/10.4103%2F0973-1229.33001.

CHAPTER 9

". . . ills that flesh is heir to."
> This is an allusion to Hamlet's famous "To Be or Not To Be" Soliloquy: Shakespeare, *Hamlet*, Act 3, Scene 1, https://tinyurl.com/wwlsgb2.

"We strive to put away from us . . ."
> Norman Macleod, "Late with Fear" *Poetry* 41, no. 3 (December 1932): 149, https://tinyurl.com/srnuwbn.

"Terror / is all I am."

   Annie Stenzel, "An Incantation for the Small Hours of the Night," *Academic Medicine* 82, no. 3 (March 2007): 290, http://doi.org/10.1097/ACM.0b013e3180309453.

. . . the anxieties many suffer . . .

   "Anxiety and Physical Illness," Harvard Women's Health Watch, Harvard Health Publishing, last modified May 9, 2018, https://tinyurl.com/rl23wm3.

Or Wendell Berry's lovely poem . . .

   Wendell Berry, "The Peace of Wild Things," Collected Poems 1957-1982 (San Francisco: Northpoint Press, 1984), p. 69.

. . . what Susan Sontag called "the kingdom of the sick."

   Susan Sontag, "Illness as Metaphor," New York Review of Books, January 26, 1978, https://tinyurl.com/swsgr56.

". . . where do you find comfort or hope in this time of illness?"

   Thomas R. McCormick, D.Min. "Spirituality and Medicine," *Ethics in Medicine*, University of Washington School of Medicine, April 2014, https://tinyurl.com/su5pyj2.

CHAPTER 10

It continues with painful images of a woman lying "half-speechless, incontinent . . ."

   Denise Levertov, "Death Psalm: Lord of Mysteries," in *Life in the Forest* (New York: New Directions, 1978).

"Let it come, as it will . . ."

   Kenyon, "Let Evening Come," 213.

". . .human merely being . . ."
e. e. cummings, "i thank You God for most this amazing," in *Xaipe* (New York: Oxford University Press, 1950), https://tinyurl.com/qvhcfmj.

CHAPTER 11

"Medication, surgery, and radiation are the weapons with which conventional medicine foolishly shoots the messengers called symptoms."
Mokokoma Mokhonoana, Twitter post, March 7, 2019. Mokokoma Mokhonoana (@Mokokoma), "#Quotes #Quotations #Aphorism #Aphorisms #QuoteOfTheDay #Made MeThink #MadeMeLaugh," Twitter, March 7, 2019, 3:47 a.m., https://tinyurl.com/uva7de5.

"I have to laugh when people ask me if I do alternative, herbal, or holistic medicine."
Sherry A. Rogers, *Detoxify or Die* (Prestige Pub, 2002), https://tinyurl.com/tobsvd6.

"When you drink ayahuasca, and you get to see divinity, you can almost never speak of it because it's too big for words."
Gerard Armond Powell, Sh*t the Moon Said: A Story of Sex, Drugs, and Ayahuasca (Health Communications, Inc., 2018).

". . . Many of those in the medical fraternity instantly label treatments in the traditional, natural or holistic health fields as quackery."
James and Lance Morcan, *The Orphan Conspiracies: 29 Conspiracy Theories from The Orphan Trilogy* (Bay of Plenty, New Zealand: Sterling Gate Books, 2014), location 2490, Kindle.

". . . Seventy-two of eighty-three Nobel Laureates in science and medicine all implicated intuition in their success."

> Keisha Blair, "How to Develop Your Intuition: Learn the 4 Steps from History's Greatest!" FinerMinds, August 12, 2017, https://tinyurl.com/v8zo6k3.

"The use of 'natural' as a synonym for 'good' is almost certainly a product of our profound alienation from the natural world."

> Eula Biss, *On Immunity: An Inoculation* (Minneapolis: Graywolf Press, 2015), 40.

CHAPTER 12

". . . 56 percent of US adults attribute financial hardships to medical costs."

> Jeff Lagasse, "Medical Costs Create Hardships for More Than Half of Americans," *Healthcare Finance*, May 2, 2019, https://tinyurl.com/tufg6nn.

So here we still are—ranking near the bottom of industrialized countries in health . . .

> Sally C. Pipes, "Does America Really Have the Worst Health System in the Developed World?" Pacific Research Institute, June 17, 2018, https://tinyurl.com/tm6pcqm.

". . . The soaring cost of health care has become the greatest threat to the long-term solvency of most advanced nations."

> Gawande, *Being Mortal*, 153.

"The poor are the ones who can never afford to have any bad luck."

> Gary A. Haugen and Victor Boutros, *The Locust Effect: Why the End of Poverty Requires the End of Violence* (New York: Oxford University Press, 2015), 146.

"On the surface, it seems odd that an interest rate can be determined by the condition of an apartment . . ."

David K. Shipler, *The Working Poor: Invisible in America* (New York: Vintage, 2008), 26.

"The pharmaceutical industry overall spends about twice as much on marketing and promotion as it does on research and development."

Ben Goldacre, *Bad Pharma: How Drug Companies Mislead Doctors and Harm Patients* (New York: Farrar, Straus and Giroux, 2014), 307.

". . . immunize yourself from the drug companies' efforts to convince you that you desperately need their advertised products."

John Abramson, MD, *Overdosed America: The Broken Promise of American Medicine* (New York: Harper Perennial, 2008), 257.

CHAPTER 13

"Music can be a powerful adjunct to the healing process."

Allan J. Hamilton, MD, *The Scalpel and the Soul: Encounters with Surgery, the Supernatural, and the Healing Power of Hope* (New York: TarcherPerigee, 2009), 226.

"Harmony, which has motions akin to the revolutions of the Soul within us . . ."

Athanasios Dritsas, "Music Therapy in Ancient Greece," Greece Is, January 9, 2017, https://tinyurl.com/smskomu.

". . . The poets did well to conjoin music and medicine . . ."

Francis Bacon, *The Oxford Francis Bacon IV: The Advancement of Learning* (New York: Clarendon Press, 2000), 203.

Recent studies have shown that chants . . .

Paul Haider, MD, "14 Proven Scientific Health Benefits of Chanting," accessed May 19, 2019, https://tinyurl.com /voaghtf.

". . . A good song is like a good meal—I just want to inhale it and then share a bite with someone else."

Hoda Kotb, *Hoda: How I Survived War Zones, Bad Hair, Cancer, and Kathie Lee* (New York: Simon and Schuster, 2011), 156.

". . . continuous musical line of our minds, the unstoppable humming."
Danielle Ofri, *What Doctors Feel: How Emotions Affect the Practice of Medicine* (Boston: Beacon Press, 2014), 3.

As poet Richard Wilbur put it . . .

Richard Wilbur, "The Eye," in *Collected Poems 1943–2004* (Orlando: Harcourt, 2006), 132.

CHAPTER 14

"The skills I learned studying fine arts in college are invaluable to me now as a physician."

"An Artful Approach to Medicine," Association of American Medical Colleges, accessed February 10, 2020, https:// tinyurl.com/up6bxy5.

All of them are taking at least a few steps to acknowledge the role of the arts in healing.

See for instance Neha Mukunda et al., "Visual Art Instruction in Medical Education: A Narrative Review," Medical Education Online 24, no. 1 (February 2019): 2–7, https://doi .org/10.1080/10872981.2018.1558657; Khullar, "What Doctors Can Learn from Looking at Art"; and Katrina A.

Bramstedt, "The Use of Visual Arts as a Window to Diagnosing Medical Pathologies," *AMA Journal of Ethics* 18, no. 8 (August 2016): 843–54, https://doi.org/10.1001/journalofethics.2016.18.8.imhl1-1608.

"It's protecting and maintaining students' empathy . . ."
Casey Lesser, "Why Med Schools Are Requiring Art Classes," Artsy, August 21, 2017, https://tinyurl.com/y7cpoa8p.

A sizeable gallery of art by patients and caregivers, including doctors and nurses, is available on the internet.
Easy access to visual art, as well as film and literature related to medicine, and illness is available at the Literature, Arts, and Medicine Database (LitMed): https://tinyurl.com/sd3gahn.

". . . Cancer Cell No. 19 . . ."
Angela Hopkins, *Cancer Cell No. 19*, 2010, acrylic on canvas with crochet circles and string, 10 x 10 inches, https://tinyurl.com/yx54ynby.

. . . Tim Lowly's stirring paintings of his daughter Temma . . .
Tim Lowly, "Temma Is a Great and Utterly Innocent Mystery," On Art and Aesthetics, March 12, 2018, https://tinyurl.com/ruqgush.

Look at Alice Neel's Works Progress Administration portraits . . .
A comment on one of these can be found at LitMed here, https://tinyurl.com/uzz9zkt.

Professionals who work to bring arts and medicine together have determined . . .
Brooke Seidelmann, "Art Can Help Patients Heal," HuffPost, November 12, 2012, https://tinyurl.com/ty2e22s.

CHAPTER 15

"We know ourselves to be made from this earth."
Susan Griffin, "Matter (How We Know)," Faith House Manhattan, January 14, 2011, https://tinyurl.com/rwfk3a3.

"The atoms of our bodies . . ."
Cami Rosso, "Are We Made of Stardust?" BBN Times, October 21, 2018, https://tinyurl.com/ub3azhl.

"A nation that destroys its soil destroys itself . . ."
Franklin D. Roosevelt, "Letter to All State Governors on a Uniform Soil Conservation Law," February 26, 1937, https://tinyurl.com/ue3vpu9.

". . . Forests are the 'lungs' of our land, purifying the air and giving fresh strength to our people."
Franklin D. Roosevelt, "Roosevelt to the Society of American Foresters," January 29, 1935, https://tinyurl.com/wbvag37.

". . . To be healed we must come with all the other creatures to the feast of Creation."
Wendell Berry and Norman Wirzba, *The Art of the Commonplace: The Agrarian Essays of Wendell Berry* (Berkeley, CA: Counterpoint, 2003), 99.

". . . Time in nature is not leisure time . . ."
Richard Louv, *Last Child in the Woods: Saving Our Children from Nature-Deficit Disorder* (Chapel Hill, NC: Algonquin, 2008), 120.

". . . Man's heart away from nature becomes hard."
Chief Luther Standing Bear, "Luther Standing Bear," IndigenousPeople.net, https://tinyurl.com/rn7cfyp.

". . . distracted from distraction by distraction."
T. S. Eliot, "Burnt Norton," 5.

". . . God uses broken things."
Vance Havner, in "Wisdom for the Heart," Wisdom Online,
November 13, 2018, https://tinyurl.com/tzxxhwe.